The Disappearing Male

The Disappearing Male

Joan Lachkar, PhD

JASON ARONSON
Lanham • Boulder • New York • Toronto • Plymouth, UK

Published by Jason Aronson
A wholly owned subsidiary of The Rowman & Littlefield Publishing Group, Inc.
4501 Forbes Boulevard, Suite 200, Lanham, Maryland 20706
www.rowman.com

10 Thornbury Road, Plymouth PL6 7PP, United Kingdom

British Library Cataloguing in Publication Information Available

Library of Congress Cataloging-in-Publication Data

Lachkar, Joan.
The disappearing male / Joan Lachkar.
p. cm.
Includes bibliographical references and index.
ISBN 978-0-7657-0909-7 (cloth : alk. paper) — ISBN (invalid) 978-0-7657-0910-3 (electronic)
1. Men—Mental health. 2. Men—Psychology. 3. Man woman relationships—Psychological aspects.
4. Psychotherapy. I. Title.
RC451.4.M45L33 2013
616.89'140811—dc23
2012036897

The paper used in this publication meets the minimum requirements of American National Standard for Information Sciences Permanence of Paper for Printed Library Materials, ANSI/NISO Z39.48-1992.

Printed in the United States of America

Love to My Family

Contents

Acknowledgments

I have learned the true meaning of mirroring and empathic attunement by working with my superb UCLA personal assistants, Marko Perko III, Crystal Lu, and Khathy Hoang, to whom I give much gratitude for their consistent support and "right on" feedback. I am also grateful to my many friends and colleagues whose encouragement was crucial in assuring me of the scholarly endeavor of writing on a topic that could easily have been relegated to the self-help rack. Included are my good friends and colleagues Vera Hamilton, Irene Fruchkbaum, Lina Suckov, Laurence Rose, Roberta Rinaldi, Rochelle Booth, Adrian Morgan, Jamie Glazov, Norman Simms, and the late Dr. Shelley Ventura. Endless appreciation to Lloyd deMause, editor of *The Journal of Psychohistory*, and a special tribute to my good friend and colleague Nancy Kobrin, whose collaboration as political analyst and scholar has greatly enhanced my work on cross-cultural topics.

Of course, there are the great masters, Drs. Otto Kernberg, James Grotstein, Albert Mason, Marvin Osman, Professor Peter Berton, Sam Vaknin, and many others whose contributions have been most valuable. I am most grateful to my family and daughters, Sharon Stone, Dr. Pamela Brody, and Nicole Raphael. Appreciation also to Peggi Ridgeway, my computer analyst and website specialist.

I thank my amazing editors Jason Aronson, Amy King, Lindsey Porambo, Melissa McNitt, and all those at Jason Aronson whose creativity and quick eye have patiently fine-tuned this work, and for their willingness to allow me to stray beyond the bounds of psychoanalysis into the world of creativity, culture, and mastery. Finally, a special tribute to my manuscript editor, Joanne Freeman, not only for her sharp eye and endless red markups but as someone who shares my artistic bent. Most of all, I am endlessly grateful to the many women (and men) who have shared their stories and whose progress and development are role models for all of us.

Introduction

. . . because happiness is not an ideal of reason but of imagination.

—Emanuel Kant

This book, based on my personal, clinical, and professional experience, was motivated by the plight of a number of women I see in my clinical practice who have been wooed, charmed, and lured, then vastly confused by what I refer to as the "Disappearing Male." Essentially, the emotional intensity of these women was the inspiration behind this book. For the past several years, I have been overwhelmed by a plethora of emails and messages from women all over the world who have been hurt and abandoned, either physically or emotionally, by men who suddenly withdrew. They wanted to find more in-depth answers. Their stories are similar and quite familiar: They involve men who at the onset appear to be madly in love and suddenly vanish without an explanation. These women cannot seem to make sense of what has occurred and need to know they are not alone and are not crazy. Getting sucked in by a Don Juan type can happen to even the most highly evolved women, including professional women from all walks of life. They come to my office confused, depressed, and traumatized by men who promise them the world and act as though the women are the love of their life—then suddenly, no call, no response.

It is noteworthy that even though this book focuses on what I term Disappearing Male Syndrome (DMS), one cannot disregard men who have legitimate reasons to disappear (physical/emotional abuse, most often the result of involvement with destructive borderline women). In addition, although this book focuses mainly on men, chapter 10 addresses the Disappearing Woman Syndrome (DWS).

Most authors have written about this subject largely from a self-help perspective and their work has been mainly aimed at women; however, a few have offered a more in-depth, analytic approach to this topic. Others may refer to the various disorders in the broad sense but do not acknowledge the specific defenses operative around emotional or physical withdrawal, as categorized in this book. We as therapists must pay meticulous attention not only to the red flags (as subtle or obvious as they may be) but must help women trust their perceptions. Because women are the bearers of children, they have a remarkable inborn capacity to perceive and read their infant's "nonverbal" communication and need to be encouraged to pay attention and listen more closely to the nonverbal cues of others—to trust what they instinctively "know." In this book I aspire to help women (and men) recognize and detect the danger signs to prevent them from faltering in their relationships and dating efforts from the onset.

This book delineates the defenses, psychodynamics, behaviors, and characteristics of eight different types of disappearing males—with the caveat that these categories are not clear and distinct entities but rather tend to vacillate back and forth. For example, both the narcissist and the obsessive-compulsive show coldness and indifference. However, while the obsessive may show coldness, he still displays feelings of social, political, or cultural concern and will spend endless time obsessing about these concerns. On the other hand, the narcissist may only show concern for his own self-serving purposes (Kernberg 1975).

Disappearing Male Syndrome is not a new concept and has deep psychological, as well as historical and cultural, significance. This work is a logical extension of my previous work, with an entirely new spotlight, different focus, and different characters. Although I do extract concepts, ideas, and theoretical formulations from my previous publications, this book differs in that the focus is specifically on the symptoms and mechanisms of defense—such as withdrawal, isolation, abandonment, anxiety, splitting, and projective identification. These types of defenses are the viruses that infect and trespass on the capacity to maintain healthy love relations. It didn't take me long to discover that one cannot examine the vicissitudes of love relations without examining the aspects of aggression, cruelty, sadism, and envy lurking in the shadows of love and intimacy.

Over the years, my pivotal work has been on *The Narcissistic/Borderline Couple* (2004), which describes what happens when a narcissist and a borderline get together in a marital bond or "bind," and how each stirs up unresolved, unconscious issues in the other and tends to identify or over-identify with the other's negative projections. I refer to this as "the dance" (between shame, blame, and guilt). I realized from this work that there are many different kinds of narcissists and many different kinds of borderlines, each of whom needs his or her own form of communication. Masterson's

(1981) groundbreaking work confirmed the importance of communication: with narcissists the therapist interprets; with borderlines the therapist confronts. In both incidences the therapist must address the vulnerability, the injury to the narcissist's omnipotent-self, and the two sides of the borderline's personality (one that loves and the other that attacks, destroys, sabotages). Heinz Kohut (1977) clearly addressed the importance of empathic understanding and how to be attuned to narcissistic patients. This inspired me to write my next two publications, *How to Talk to a Narcissist* (2008b) and *How to Talk to a Borderline* (2011). Addressing the need for an effective way to communicate with both narcissists and borderlines led to my devising two languages—The Language of Empathology for the narcissist and The Language of Dialectics for the borderline.

Throughout this book I revisit the various couples and topics from my previous works, including early trauma and past archaic injuries and the area where they interface. I refer to this as the vertex of vulnerability, or *The V-Spot* (2008a), the most sensitive area of emotional vulnerability that becomes aroused when one partner hits a raw spot or pushes the other's buttons. I find the term "V-spot" far more accessible than the psychoanalytic term "archaic injury," and most patients respond to it more readily. *My boyfriend really pushed my V-spot when he said I needed to lose weight!*

Drawing mainly from psychoanalysis, social psychology, and psychohistory and using a metapsychological approach to study individuals, couples, and groups—including those across cultures—I have had to endure many criticisms claiming that we as psychoanalysts have no business analyzing other cultures. However, within today's vast and ever-changing clinical practices, which embrace people from various cultures and ethnic groups, mental health professionals are now beginning to understand not only that the dynamics of people vary from culture to culture, but also that the degree of governmental abuses and violations against women vary across cultures. *In my country it is okay to beat our wives when they don't obey!*

Another challenge we face when discussing these disorders is: Which theorist do we adhere to? When we talk about narcissists and borderlines, to whose narcissist or whose borderline are we referring? A Freudian narcissist? A Kleinian narcissist? A Kernbergian or Kohutian narcissist? What kind of a borderline? A Kernbergian borderline, a Masterson borderline, or borderline as conceived by a more contemporary theorist, such as Marsha Linehan?

Even though there are many variations on the theme of disappearance, the major defenses are withdrawal, isolation, splitting, disassociation, and corresponding ways of retreating from love, closeness, intimacy, and commitment—the big "C." The goal of this book is to inform and guide therapists to help their patients deal with loss, trauma, and betrayal over the sudden abandonment by an intimate partner or lover. It also has significance for the awareness and self-esteem of women in the dating world. While myriad self-help books exist, few take on the voice of a professional psychotherapist. Women today are extraordinarily well read, sophisticated, well analyzed, psychologically minded, and appreciate a more in-depth approach. This book provides the necessary tools to help these women disengage from the negative projections with which they internalize and identify. Recognizing these subjective areas and understanding how the least little thing can trigger someone's V-spot or archaic injury can be most beneficial for women who are trying to heal from falling for a man who supplied them with dreams and promises and then vanished. It is comforting for these women to know that the men who have disappeared usually are not withdrawing from them but from a part of themselves that cannot tolerate the state of intimacy or vulnerability (Thorsen 2010). Each pathology described in this book has its own unique style of withdrawing. The way a narcissist vanishes when feeling injured is different from the way a schizoid vanishes when feeling suffocated, or an obsessive-compulsive vanishes when confronted with emotionality.

Donald Gilmore (2001) wrote a popular book about *the misogynist male* (from the Greek word meaning "woman hater") that was a composite of all men lumped into one and shed insight into the prototypical man who controls, dominates, sabotages, or sees women as all good or all bad. However, it failed to recognize the qualitative distinctions operative within misogyny: e.g., a narcissistic misogynist, one who has feelings of superiority over the women; a borderline misogynist, who envies the woman and therefore must destroy her; or a schizoid misogynist, who can make initial contact with a woman and then totally disassociate.

The organizing principle of this book is to examine and describe a variety of personality disorders and symptoms under the rubric of the disappearing male that women familiarly encounter, in a way that is user friendly. The symptoms and dynamics outlined in this book are designed to enhance an individual's capacity to become aware of pitfalls involved in dealing with men who have Disappearing Male Syndrome (DMS). To that end each chapter includes vignettes and case examples that help women understand the abandonment scenarios that they will most frequently encounter.

Writing this book has also entailed noting the equality, or inequality, between the sexes. I have been grappling with the view of the male as being more inclined than the female to avoid issues around intimacy, dependency, vulnerability attachment, and to display differences in his bonding experiences. Thus, the focus is primarily on the Disappearing Male Syndrome, not Disappearing Partner Syndrome.

THE CHAPTERS

Chapter 1 contains a definition and overview of the disappearing male, discusses the defense mechanisms involved, and touches on societal and cultural influences related to the American Dream fantasy and the problems of living up to it. This chapter also discusses materialism, wealth, the changing views on marriage, declining marriage rates, blended families, single parent homes, gay marriages, sexual liberation, and the increasing number of women in the workforce. Chapter 2 revisits and introduces the classical theoretical approaches and acknowledges some of the more contemporary ones that have been most influential in shaping this book. It also addresses the confusion and overlap resulting from the many variations on the theme of the disappearing male.

The following chapters cover the various types of disappearing male. Chapter 3 introduces the disappearing narcissist, described and defined as the entitlement lover who is quick to withdraw either physically or emotionally when narcissistically injured. Included in the different types of narcissists in this category is the Narcissistic Artist, who relentlessly makes his art the number one priority in his life. Chapter 4 describes the disappearing borderline—defined as the destructive, envious, manipulative, clingy, and seductive man who bonds/fuses with his objects and when feeling betrayed or abandoned will seek revenge, attack, or retaliate. Chapter 6 focuses on the obsessive-compulsive disappearing male, who is more concerned with objects then emotions. Chapter 7 resurrects the passive-aggressive disorder, which has been removed from the DSM IV, and categorizes him as disappearing into dependency mode. Chapter 8 examines the depressive disappearing male, who uses his depression for victimization, self-pity, and self-hatred turned inward.

Chapter 9 discusses the cross-cultural aspects of the disappearing male, ranging from the domestic to the global, examining how religion, traditions, ideology, and child-rearing practices foster certain patterns of behavior in men that impact the treatment of women. Chapter 10 tackles the subject of the disappearing woman–someone who is cold, aloof, withdrawn, and indifferent. At the other end of the spectrum is the woman who is consumed with emotionality, overreacts, cries easily, acts out impulsively and provocatively, and when ignored or not given what she considers sufficient attention becomes shamelessly violent and crude. *I don't care what you think of me. I only exist for your love!* Chapter 11 offers treatment techniques, procedures, and suggestions for both therapists and patients dealing with this Houdini syndrome (DMS).

Chapter 12 presents closing thoughts and reflections on timely topics that help us adapt our clinical practices to changes taking place around us. This book would not be complete without making reference to the new way people meet and interact. Social networking and Internet dating has exploded in recent years. Thus, this chapter looks at prototypical profiles and profile names (disguised, of course) and shows how therapists can guide their patients into noting the danger signs and decoding email messages. It also provides techniques to sharpen listening skills.

While this book is designed for the mental health profession, it extends beyond that to appeal to the motivated, intelligent woman who wants to get back on an even keel after a disturbing encounter with a vanishing male, and to guard against finding herself in this situation again and again—what Freud would refer to as a repetitive compulsion (Freud 1920).

Most of all, this book was written with the hope that it will prove beneficial to all those struggling with the complexities and madness inherent in love relations.

Chapter One

Now You See Him, Now You Don't

Defining the disappearing male is no easy task because of the myriad facets involved. There are at least two ways to approach the definition. First, the most common scenario involves a male who purports to be madly in love then suddenly disappears without any explanation. "I'll call you!" he says. But you don't hear a word. Poof. He's gone! Second, it is important to note that disappearance does not necessarily constitute a physical withdrawal; it may also be an emotional withdrawal (avoidance, detachment, splitting, gaslighting, deafening silence, isolation), which can even be more puzzling and painful to his partner. The self-absorbed narcissist, the workaholic obsessive-compulsive, and the "out-to-lunch" robotic schizoid often fit into these categories. *He never listens to me. Whenever I ask him what he would like to do or what he wants for dinner, his typically stoic response is that he doesn't know or doesn't care! And if I pursue it further, he gets mad at me for nagging.*

As many of us know, just as a man's attention and devotion can make a woman ecstatically happy, they can also bring the woman to the edge of madness. The not knowing, not having any finality or closure leaves the woman with only the fantasy, and a false sense of what could have been, should have been. Self-persecution is a common affective experience among these women: *Where did I go wrong? Was it my fault?* Often they are blindsided by men who present such an exquisite false self that they could dupe even the most seasoned therapist.

Unknowingly, the women enter into the relationship with idealization and grandiose expectations and do not see the man for who he really is. *I should have known better!* Some of these men, who often are jaded, bring into a budding relationship trauma and fears that disrupt the potentiality of a healthy love bond. What is even worse is the final "poof" and the need to deal with the unfulfilled dream left behind. Women who have been loved and cherished and experience a loss cope better than women left with an unfilled dream. *I was so close to getting what I have been longing for my whole life.* To paraphrase the oft-quoted adage, it's better to have been loved and lost than never to have been loved at all.

At first, I wasn't sure I was attracted to him. He kept pursuing me until one day I decided that this guy really likes me and I would give him a chance. We did not share many common interests. I liked the arts, and he preferred sports. Nevertheless he got along with my family, and always brought presents to my family when was invited. He was very successful, a well-to-do businessman, and seemingly a good family man type. I did not pay too much attention to the fact that he had been married four times and complained that each of his wives "took him to the cleaners." One had an affair, and the others "used" him, practically bankrupting him through their lavish spending habits. There were endless custody and alimony battles. He said, "Even though I lost everything to those bitches, I was able to rebuild myself." What I didn't realize was that I had a man who was jaded, had been raked over the coals, and who brought into our relationship his "used baggage." He appreciated that I loved to cook, and that I did not need to go to five-star hotels and restaurants.

Throughout our relationship he kept telling me how much he appreciated me, how different I was. He acted as though I was the only woman he could ever love and trust. He continued to smother me with the gifts, made plans and reservations, and even took me to operas and concerts, which he basically had no interest in. He continually told me I was the love of his life. Everything was good until about a year later when I decided to talk about commitment. The next morning I walked outside of my house to get my newspaper and there on my doorstep were all the belongings and overnight things that I kept at his place for when I stayed over. Not a word since! What did I do? Was I too demanding? Getting too old? Was there another woman? I was in shock. There was no note, no calls, nothing. I called and called, but to no avail. He refused to answer my calls, and I ultimately got a text message asking me never to contact him again. I can only assume that because he was married four times that the "C" word must have really hit him. I was devastated. I guess I will never know why he left.

Never before has disappearing male syndrome been so prevalent—leaving in its wake a growing segment of women who have been traumatized by the sudden withdrawal of their love partner. One could speculate that men today are products of the women's movement, sexual freedom, liberation, being raised in single-family homes, the loosening of morality and ethics. They are also products of the "me–me" society peopled with overly preoccupied and self-absorbed types. The most common advice given to women, mainly by pop book writers, is to reverse the chase: "Let the man come after you. Let him wait a few days before calling him back. Let him suffer!" Unfortunately, this advice basically has no pertinence in the situation involving the disappearing male.

Another rationale for the increasing incidence of the disappearing male is to view men as hunters pre-programmed for the chase, geared for conquest and challenge, and for winning the prize. Today men can easily get what they want without taking on the responsibility of marriage. Women have provided an open door policy that encourages living together—*Let's try it out*—making it easy for men to win the prize without breaking a sweat, so to speak. Some say it goes against man's primal instinct to procreate with only one female.

Yet another reason for men's disappearing act includes fear of domination by today's more independent women, who can fend for themselves and are in direct contrast to the more "traditional" women who expect and depend on the man to provide for them. Additionally, the fear of failure looms large among the male population. High divorce rates, previous failed marriages, financial and custody battles all have a significant impact on the choice to run from commitment.

Although all of the above reasons have credibility and certainly do occur in the ebb and flow of love relations, they do not spring from a psychoanalytic approach. My basic premise is that the majority of men described in this book are inclined toward mental and characterological disorders. Beyond the hunter–gatherer theories are mature men who (1) have never overcome unresolved oedipal issues and mastery over their oedipal rivals, (2) have never separated-individuated from the maternal object—i.e., fusion with the mother, (3) fear vulnerability, believing that with commitment come dependency and feelings of smallness, entrapment, engulfment, and suffocation—which draws them away from the love object for fear that they'll be sucked into a black hole, (4) see the woman as a part object, not as a woman with needs, feelings, desires, and concerns but as an object solely designed to meet and satisfy his self-serving needs—*Ask not what you can do for the woman, but what she can do for you!*, (5) confuse reality and fantasy—*At the time I wanted marriage, but when I thought of what it entails, I changed my mind*, (6) have sadistic, aggressive, anal impulses and keep the woman on hold, always waiting, and in a continual state of deprivation.

Furthermore, there are the defense mechanisms, splitting, projection, projective identification, and envy. *No one gave anything to me so why should I give anything to you?* Imagine how big and powerful a narcissist feels when a woman begs and pleads for commitment. It fuels his narcissistic needs to have a woman so desirous of him. The more needy and desperate she is, the more she coats his protective, shielding armor, and the more he withdraws and isolates himself. Just imagine the same man giving in and agreeing to commit. Suddenly he feels reduced to a state of nothingness, smallness, dependency, vulnerability—not the best casting role for a narcissist, especially when he feels injured. By contrast, the healthy man has a different voice: "I want to find the love of my life and settle down. I'm tired of all this running around." Of course, the voice of Freud chimes in, "The job of women is to tame men."

Many of the women left behind have spent countless hours in sessions ruminating about what they did wrong, blaming and persecuting themselves. It is noteworthy that although these "sudden" disappearances occur on different levels and during different time periods—it could be the first encounter, or a few dates, or weeks, months, or even years, apart—the women left behind may all feel the same hurt and pain. *He picked me up on the first date. We knew right away the chemistry was there. He said he could not wait until our next date. He mentioned taking me places he envisioned for us to travel to together. He kissed me gently and said he would call. I never heard a word from him again.*

Therapists need to be on the lookout for those displaying or dealing with the effects of DMS, mainly the woman's proclivity to blame herself, and her incapacity to tolerate and live in the state of not knowing. No matter how emotionally stable the woman is, this kind of experience can be earth shattering—although women with more self-esteem are less inclined toward self-blame and self-persecution and tend to heal faster than those with less ego strength. No matter how the woman may feel she failed or what wrongdoings she may have contributed to the relationship (e.g., making too many demands, being too critical, nagging too much, feeling too needy), there is never an excuse for a man who has had more than just a few casual dates to bail out without processing the experience with the women he was "in love" with.

HOW THE MEN FEEL

There are men who admit that as soon as they get a sense of approaching danger (entrapment, suffocation, dependency), they're gone. For many it is an unmentalized experience. *I don't think; I just feel! Just give me my space!* Many women report that things can go along fairly smoothly until the word commitment comes up. Often this is the trigger that makes men flee. Many men confess that they don't want commitment and are happy with the way things are, with just dating or cohabitation. Some admit that as soon as they hear or even think about the "C" word, they feel suffocated, closed in, and seek space. Others admit they no longer feel the excitement that they felt when they first started dating. They feel the relationship has become boring, that the woman has become too demanding, or that they do not want to provide for a woman who is not financially secure.

I was getting bored. I just wanted to go out and meet other women and get laid. She wanted commitment, a baby. I already have two kids. At this stage of my life I don't need a relationship. I can order take-out, go on my boat, see my buddies, and have a great time! I tried to give her the message that I was losing interest. Couldn't she sense that? Instead she kept nagging me about why I didn't hold her hand, why I stopped calling as frequently as I used to. At first I was very attracted to her, but as soon as she started to do the pressure thing about commitment, I freaked out. I guess I stayed because I had a lot of ambivalence. Part of me wants to be a nice guy. I didn't want to hurt or disappoint her, so I just kept afloat. It didn't bother me that her biological clock was running out. I felt that was her issue to deal with, not mine. I guess I was living like I was someone else, not my real self. So I just packed my bags and left. And now I can be free.

Let us take a moment to see what the response might be from a mentally healthy man.

Gee, honey. It's been over two years that we have been together, and I don't feel that our relationship is really moving forward the way you want it to, and I am not ready to commit. I know this is painful, and this is not intended to hurt you. What I suggest we do is go to some couples therapy and spell out our issues. Right now I don't see a future together, but at least we will have an opportunity to sort out our issues and be able to talk to someone who can help us sort things out.

Men frequently resort to the view of "never again," even though these men are merely deluding themselves that they are protecting themselves from entrapment. This is especially true of those men who have not adequately overcome their oedipal conflicts or who have been hurt, used, and misused by women—most commonly after a divorce in which they feel that not only the women but the legal system has raked them over the coals. The therapeutic challenge in treating these men is threefold. First to identify their feelings; second to trace the origins of an early experience (e.g., mother overly possessive, controlling, and domineering), or the original archaic injury or V-spot; third, to clarify and sort out how they are bringing old baggage to a budding relationship.

THE V-SPOT

The "V-Spot" (Lachkar 2008a) is an essential link drawing together the defenses that get pummeled in relational love bonds. It is a term I originated to reflect and redefine Heinz Kohut's (1971, 1977) narcissistic injury—our most sensitive area of vulnerability that gets stirred up when one person hits an emotional chord in another person. It is the heart of our most fragile self, an area of emotional sensitivity known as the archaic injury, a product of early trauma that one holds onto throughout one's life. The V-spot is a zone that is triggered by any threat or reminder of this early trauma, of not being special or the "only one." I found the term V-spot to be more user friendly than archaic injury, because it helps pinpoint the nature of the reaction produced. It is the emotional counterpart of the G-spot. The G-spot is purely physical, whereas the V-spot is purely emotional. With provocation of the V-spot comes a loss of one's sense of self. Everything gets shaken, and ego fragmentation ensues (Lachkar 2008a, 2008b).

Examples of V-spot reactions:

Why do you serve your brother first when he comes for dinner? I am your husband. I should come before him!

Every time I see a photo of her ex-boyfriend I go ballistic! Then we get into a fight!

THE NARCISSISTIC/BORDERLINE RELATIONSHIP

In my book *The Narcissistic/Borderline Couple* (Lachkar 2004b), I described this as a beleaguered relationship between two developmentally arrested people who coerce each other into playing certain roles. I single out this pairing here because it is the relationship that most often highlights the disappearing male syndrome. Both the narcissist and borderline bring into their current relationships their unresolved archaic selves, experiences embedded in old sentiments. These two personality types enter into a psychological dance, and consciously or unconsciously stir up in each other highly charged feelings (their V-spots) rooted in early unresolved conflicts. The reality is that each partner needs the other to play out his or her own personal relational drama. Together they engage in a dance that is ongoing, circular, never ending. Each stirs up the other's painful injuries without ever reaching any conflict resolution (Lachkar 1992, 2004b, 2008a, 2008b, 2010).

There are many different types of narcissists and many different types of borderlines. Each type has its own operating system of defenses groomed to impede love and intimacy. Each one needs a special form of communication.

The way one talks to a narcissist is quite different than how one would talk to a borderline; thus, I devised the Language of Empathology for the narcissist and the Language of Dialectics for the borderline (see chapter 2). I consider the V-spot to be an essential tool for understanding the traumatic impact one partner has upon the other partner. Although it sometimes seems to be the case, narcissists and borderlines do not undergo special training on how to become a narcissist or borderline; however, they seem to share a similar operating system of defenses within an intrapsychic and interpersonal world. One wrong word and they blow! The following is an example of the dance between a narcissist and a borderline and their corresponding V-spots:

Woman: *I want to get married!*

Man: *Married! Why do you need to get married?*

W: *Just living together isn't enough.*

M: *But it is as though we are already married.*

W: *But we are not married.*

M: *Marriage is just a piece of paper.*

W: *It is not just a piece paper.*

M: *I was married before and it is no different than now.*

W: *Then why did you get divorced?*

M: *Because I didn't want to stay married.*

W: *But if it was just a piece of paper why did you get a divorce?*

M: *If you don't stop badgering me, I'm going to pack up and leave.*

W: *So leave as you always do you whenever we have this discussion.*

M: *Well, I don't want to get married.*

W: *Then you do admit it is more than a piece of paper! It's a commitment.*

M: *You still have plenty of time to have a baby, so you need to stop pressuring me about marriage!*

The case that follows involves a narcissistic/borderline couple (Lachkar 2004b). It incorporates and illustrates some of the techniques and methods I revisit throughout this book. This includes reference to the use of the language of empathology for the narcissist and the language of dialectics for the borderline. Both methods are designed to help the couple access their corresponding V-spots.

The Case of Janice and Jeffrey

Janice and Jeffrey have been living together for three years, and Janice is concerned that her biological clock is running out. Jeffrey (the narcissist) is a lawyer preoccupied with his work, while Janice (the borderline) is an actor seeking out roles at casting auditions.

> Therapist: *Greetings! So what brings you here?*
>
> Janice: *Jeffrey and I have been living together for three years and still there is no commitment, no marriage, and my biological clock is running out.*
>
> Jeffrey: *That's not true. It has not been three years. You stormed out so many times to stay with your mother for months.*
>
> Janice: *That has nothing to do with it. The reality is I want a ring and a commitment. He's been promising and promising and so far nothing is happening.*
>
> Jeffrey: *I told her that will happen when the time is right.*
>
> Th: (listens attentively)
>
> Janice: *Time is right for who? You? Why does everything have to be on your terms?*
>
> Jeffrey: *Because I'm the one who is working day and night making a living, and you hardly get any work except those little part-time gigs.*
>
> Th: *So what I am hearing is that you, Janice, want marriage and commitment and feel pressured because you are 41 years old, and that it is now or never. And you, Jeffrey, feel rebuked by the pressure put upon you.*
>
> Jeffrey: *Doesn't she know by now I don't respond to demands or pressure?*
>
> Th: *Maybe you can educate us. How can she express her needs?*

Jeffrey: *Needs! All I hear about from you therapists are needs! Needs! What about just going with the flow?*

Th: (does she confront him or does she instead turn to the language of empathology?) *Jeffrey, from what I know, you are a very successful and powerful attorney. Amazing how you got into one of the biggest law firms in New York. That is quite an achievement.*

Jeffrey: *Well, I'm glad you think so. Janice could care less about my work. All she thinks about is marriage and having a baby.*

Janice: *I do appreciate your work. I think you are a brilliant lawyer. I'm just unhappy.*

Jeffrey: *Well, Janice, if you are so unhappy why do you stay? You're free to leave at any time and find a guy to marry you.*

Janice: *Because I am in love with you.*

Th: (tapping into Janice's V-spot, her grandiose self that is more concerned with proving something than taking care of her own needs) *Janice, this doesn't sound like love. You are with a very high-powered, successful man, and you are trying to force him to do something he does not want to do.*

Janice: *Why doesn't he want to marry me? He certainly loves me enough to have me live with him. I guess this has been a pattern in my life, where I always fall for the unavailable man and feel that I can fix him, change him.*

Th: *Janice, I very much appreciate your insight into yourself. Now let's hear from Jeffrey. What would happen if you did marry Janice? How would you feel?*

Jeffrey: *I would feel trapped, suffocated, and weak, like a powerless little kid.*

Th: *Is that how your father felt when he married your mother?*

Jeffrey: *My mother dominated and totally controlled him. He was trapped, and I don't want to be like my father.*

Th: (tapping into Jeffrey's V-spot) *I am very impressed because I think you are telling us that you would feel vulnerable, and feeling vulnerable would be tantamount to weakness, impotency, and smallness.*

Jeffrey: *Exactly! I don't want to feel like that!*

Th: *Jeffrey, how would you react if I told you that feeling vulnerable is actually a very healthy state, and that although withdrawing makes you feel momentarily big and powerful, it is not long lasting.*

Janice: *That's what I do. I make myself vulnerable all the time and look what I get.*

Th: *Janice, you don't make yourself vulnerable. Instead of facing your real needs you become demanding. So what we have then is a dance. The more you demand the more Jeffrey withdraws from his real needs.*

Jeffrey: *I do have real needs, and I don't want to get married.*

Th: *We have to stop now, but it is hard at this stage of your relationship to make any decisions about what to do until we see what the real needs are. Jeffrey, while you withdraw from feelings of vulnerability and, Janice, while you try to fix Jeffrey, the real needs of you both get covered up with layers of protective armor, or what we call defense mechanisms. So these are some of the issues to think about, and I will see you next week.*

Janice and Jeffrey: *Thanks. Bye now*!

Discussion

The therapist, noting that Jeffrey is narcissistic, employs the language of empathology to empower him, reminding him how successful and powerful he is in preparation for introducing him to his vulnerable self, or V-spot. For Janice, the therapist uses the language of dialectics to show the splitting that occurs, revealing the two sides of her personality. One wants to get her needs met, while the other side subjugates her needs for a grandiose omnipotent self that thinks she can fix Jeffrey.

This kind of case always presents a challenge for the therapist. Before concentrating on the relationship, the therapist first tries to open up the therapeutic space to show that while these primitive defenses are operative, it is hard to know what to do. Jeffrey has a highly distorted view of what it means to be vulnerable, and Janice has the grandiose fantasy that she can "fix" Jeffrey. Yes, Janice wants commitment; but what about the commitment to herself and to her own biological clock? Yes, Jeffrey wants to stay in the relationship, but he needs to understand that one cannot love and be intimate without feelings of vulnerability.

This case illustrates the high degree of ambivalence involved and how important it is not to make any major decisions when the ego becomes dysfunctional and when defenses dominate the relationship.

SOCIETAL INFLUENCES

An examination of the disappearing male syndrome and its effect on the psychodynamics of the individual or the couple must take into consideration the environmental, societal, and cultural factors involved. Let us begin with the American Dream fantasy that many of us identify with: Everyone should be happy! But then what happens to meaning and purpose in life? The Hollywood happy-hour philosophy gives us the message that "if you are not happy, have an affair, live it up! Look at us; we are the rich and famous." How about a posh wedding like that of Kim Kardashian—marriage that lasts as long as a trip to an In and Out Burger! The government is aware that the American Dream is not so easy to attain for the poor, the underprivileged, and the unemployed and tries to compensate by providing social welfare, Medicaid, and unemployment benefits. This doesn't even touch on the other societal aspects of the American Dream that involve equal opportunity and liberty for all regardless of gender, race, and ethnicity.

Another aspect of the American Dream is that those who are not happy should just stop what they're doing and seek happiness elsewhere. The opportunities are plentiful. Fortunately, the pendulum is now starting to swing in the opposite, more realistic direction. But for many years therapists and patients focused on the nirvanic bubble as a main criterion for a relationship. Dennis Prager, talk show host and author of *Happiness Is a Serious Problem: A Human Nature Repair Manual* (1998), has some profound views on these topics. Although Prager is not a clinical psychologist and his arguments are not based on clinical studies, he is a clear thinker and his view on happiness is worth mentioning. He suggests many people should give up expectations, forget about demanding unconditional love, and should be more grounded in work and creativity as opposed to entitlement. He notes that happiness is a subjective experience.

I could not help thinking how Prager's advice is very much in accordance with Marsha Linehan's concept of Mindlessness and Acceptance (see chapter 2). It is also in concert with psychoanalytic thinking that "curing" patients to ensure happiness paradoxically is not the cure. Patients really want to find meaning and purpose in the meaningless and the chaos. My immigrant Polish–German Jewish mother defined happiness based on whether or not I ate all the food on my plate. Basically, Prager is saying that happiness is a myth. This is closely aligned to my concept that the replacement for happiness is functioning and the search for meaning and purpose.

There are many other factors that contribute to the disappearing male syndrome. The breakdown of the family began with the increase of divorce and with the rise in the number of babies born out of wedlock. This has resulted in fathers—particularly prevalent among black males—leaving their families and in women getting all sorts of free help from the government when the male leaves. Among reasons for fear of commitment are the rise of feminism, sexual freedom, drugs, alcohol, sexual addiction, the media, and porno. The way we behave is often engineered by Hollywood stars and politicians acting as our idealized role models. I might even be inclined to lay part of the blame for the increasing incidence of DMS to fast food. (*Who needs a women to cook. I can get all I need from McDonald's or Subway!*)

One of the most obvious factors that contributes to fear of commitment is anxiety about intimacy and vulnerability. Often men confuse vulnerability with impotence, smallness, and helplessness. *I feel like I've lost my balls.* Most men don't recognize that feelings of vulnerability are signs of mental health and normalcy; rather they confuse vulnerability with insecurity and low self-esteem. They replace the love object with grandiosity, omnipotence, and pomposity. *Who needs you? Look, I can do it myself! I have my own computer, my own sailboat, my Harley, my power workouts. Who needs you!* Today there is far less focus on home, family, raising children, and greater focus on self-aggrandizement, self-love, achievement, and success. Excitement is our newest addictive drug. It is imperative for therapists to address the issues of dependency as a very healthy and normal state of mind; most men have that in reverse and believe their dependency needs are pathological and that feeling needy or vulnerable means they are weak and impotent.

At the domestic level, most people in our society have the basic need to achieve success, recognition, and other forms of self-gratification. However, some have gotten carried away with the American Dream, the endless search for power, fame, recognition, and fortune. The same holds true with meeting a mate. They buy into the fantasy that they will meet the perfect man, the perfect woman who matches some idealized image that will fulfill them or make them happy. Unfortunately, this often ends in disappointment and disillusionment. Without trying to sound too narcissistic myself, as a person living in Los Angeles, the hubbub of the entertainment world, I have had a great deal of hands-on experience with these idealists. Healthy narcissism does not interfere with or damage the quality of life of those around us. Personal relations should not be regarded as a zero-sum game.

Do marital and dating relations reflect this search for success, power, money, sex, excitement, and fame as something far more pervasive than the desire to maintain an intimate love bond? Environmental stresses and strains become an epidemic in a me–me society without regard for family or community, let alone the other person. Paradoxically, the disappearing male actually becomes a victim to the very thing he tries to avoid, for he is the one who is expected to fulfill unrealistic dreams or else be equated with weakness and impotency.

DARK SIDE OF THE AMERICAN DREAM: ENTITLEMENT RUN WILD

Today we are also experiencing the dark side of the American Dream. The backlash of the American dream encompasses many factors—the fear of commitment, fear of intimacy, fear of success (unresolved oedipal issues), the feminist movement, the sexual revolution, economic factors, gender differences, changes in the institution of marriage (cohabitation/gay marriages), and cross-cultural marriages (chapter 9 discusses this in more detail). It is understandable how certain groups will form an identification not only with powerful leaders but with certain movie stars, political figures, economic moguls, or technical giants in our society that have a proclivity to act out their grandiose or omnipotent fantasies. Mother America offers a perfect template by virtue of the American Dream she has nurtured—a collective group fantasy that everyone is entitled to be recognized as superior. This has resulted in a general obsession with unlimited wealth, success, fame, power, and beauty. Thus, people in these groups consider themselves special, unique, and entitled to the best that life can offer—including other people's hard-earned money—and to only service themselves.

CEOs, executives, and millionaire moguls such as Bernard Madoff, corporate executive Samuel Waksal of IMClone, and Ken Lay of Enron are typical examples of businessmen with their own self-serving regulating system that subscribes to the collective group fantasy of entitlement and grandiose schemes, also known as malignant narcissism (Lachkar 2010; see chapter 3). We are also experiencing a society in which people have become so obsessed with success and achievement that love, intimacy, and family no longer take center stage.

FEMINISM AND GENDER DIFFERENCES

What do societal pressures and issues have to do with the disappearing male? After WWII there was a general loosening of moral standards in society. This was followed by the beginning of the sexual revolution. In the 1960s women were tossing their bras, the Woodstock phenomenon was taking off like wildfire, and sunflower women were sprouting up all over. It does not take a social scientist to figure out the effect this has on men—mainly that a man feels he does not have to commit to one woman but can flock from one to the next. Women are everywhere, plentiful and free! Then we have the women's movement and the age of feminism. Gloria Steinem advocated radicalized feminism and stressed even further the equality of men and women.

Despite the rise of feminism and the ongoing effort to ensure that women are granted equal rights in the workplace, women still fall prey to the seduction of men. Even as women become more prominent in the workforce, they eventually feel the need for marriage, a family, and begin to race against their biological clocks. The lack of empathy or concern the narcissistic man displays for his partner's needs may keep her on hold in a relationship while her clock ticks on. Stay-at-home moms often feel beleaguered because men can continue pursuing their endeavors without the disruption of menstrual cramps, kids needing to be picked up from school, menopause night sweats, and the like. This can encourage further backlash of the feminist movement in the form of divorce, with its attendant custody, alimony, and spousal support battles.

While the focus of this book is on symptoms and psychological pathogenesis, it is also noteworthy to mention that not all disappearing males exhibit these defenses. Author John Gray (1993) says it all in *Men Are from Mars, Women are from Venus*. This enormously popular—although not scientific—book outlining the different communication styles and emotional needs of the two sexes suggests that men and women function via different operating systems. Gray outlines the ways men differ from women in their responses to stress and to love and suggests that the male will withdraw or take a time out until he can come up with a way to solve a dilemma with which he is confronted. (See the reference in chapter 6 to the Robotic Male. While there is a carry-over to other disorders, this section further emphasizes how even though a man may be cut off from his feelings and emotions he will not necessarily withdraw, as does the defensive disappearing male.)

According to Kernberg (1975), masochism in personal relations is more common in women than in men. He attributes this to psychodynamic and social factors that reinforce an overall masochism in women and a tendency toward sadism in men. His findings indicate that masochistic love relations are more frequent in women, who tend to be more submissive in the workplace as well. A very common syndrome is that during adolescence young girls often fall in love with an idealized, unavailable, or deeply disappointing man, which has an influence on their future love life. Falling in love with unavailable men may lead to future romantic encounters that are not realistic and result in constant disappointment. It is noteworthy that these women may unconsciously seek unrequited lovers, which impels them to endlessly repeat the same experience—thus helping to perpetuate the disappearing male syndrome.

Feminist psychoanalyst Jessica Benjamin in *Bonds of Love* (1988) substantiates Kernberg's findings that male domination has its etiology in gender roles. Women are raised to be submissive, to be the primary caretakers, and are able to sustain identification with the mother. On the other hand, men have to repudiate the mother in order to define their independence and masculinity. Benjamin finds that many young males who are not able to work through aggression will remain forever cruel and even sadistic toward the mother and eventually to their female partners. She claims the tendency toward erotic love becomes an integral part of male domination vis-à-vis their relationships with women. This is a form of misidentifying and detaching from the mother, making her more of an object.

Talk show host Melanie Evans (2010) brings us back to the more traditional sense of gender issues, relating how women have a proclivity toward being the caretakers and nurturers, that women are more co-dependent than men, and more inclined to bear or tolerate the destructive enactments of their male narcissistic partners. Since women are the bearers of children and tend to be in tune with their infant's nonverbal communications, they make perfect prey for men who target their vulnerabilities. Men, on the other hand, are more predisposed than women to be the aggressors and to dissociate and split off from their emotions. This makes the women statistically at greater risk for abuse and victimization. Violence against women is not a new story, but we now have added a new mix to the bag: Men in the West, as well as jihadists from the Middle East, who feel sexually inadequate and threatened by powerful women, resort to controlling, domineering, and using force. The lure of this false power has big appeal for some young Western men to become jihadists and convert to Islam: *Now we are in control of our women!*

Other societal factors that encourage disappearing male syndrome are divorce and absent fathers. Men who are completely disillusioned by the relationships they have experienced often feel persecuted and fearful of engaging in new relationships. The high incidence of divorce and deadbeat dads has significantly impacted today's male. Fearful that a new relationship will create the same trauma, he is reluctant to commit to another one. He may also have been a product of divorce himself and as such may have experienced an absent father, which has further preprogrammed him to avoid intimate attachments.

MARRIAGE: SAYING "I DON'T" INSTEAD OF "I DO!"

Napoleon was convinced that marriage should not be an affair of hormones and propinquity, but of acquiring and transmitting property and conceiving and raising children. He also felt that a husband's adultery was not a cause for divorce unless the man kept his mistress under the same roof as his wife. However, he declared a wife's adultery to be grounds for divorce—even though he twice forgave Josephine for cuckolding him.

Women have no rank . . . woman was made for man, and man for the country, family. . . . We treat women too well, and in this way have spoiled everything. We have done every wrong by raising them to our level. Truly the Oriental nations have more mind and sense than we in declaring the wife to be the actual property of the husband. In fact, nature has made woman our slave. . . . Woman is given to man that she may bear children . . . consequently she is his property, just as a fruit tree is the property of the gardener.

Excerpt from *The Age of Napoleon*, Part Three (Durant & Durant 1975)

Cheating and infidelity are not new concepts. They have been around since the creation of man. But they have now become rampant. Hollywood and prime time TV have been on the leading edge of changing societal mores. An article that appeared in the *Los Angeles Times* (2011b) suggests that bed hopping on the Hollywood scene and movie and TV screens throughout the nation has contributed to the proliferation of divorce by making divorce appear more acceptable. In addition, Hollywood has given us permission to indulge in greater sexual freedom and promiscuity. Since the 1960s and 1970s, we've seen a general loosening of mores and a cultural shift away from the core values of marriage, fidelity, and monogamy.

Cynicism about marriage is rampant. According to recent statistics, of the more than one million annual marriages in California, at least one of two ends in divorce. It is no wonder that California has the highest divorce rate in the nation. It was the first state to enact a no-fault divorce law. In Los Angeles, the hub of the entertainment industry, marriages and divorces have become an integral part of show biz. They bring exposure and notoriety to those whose star might be on the wane. Kim Kardashian is a good example of this type of crocodile marriage—a lavish wedding offers a lot of mileage in media coverage. Californians are also more liberal minded and divorce is more socially acceptable than in the rest of the nation.

Is marriage becoming an endangered institution? It's ironic that what the gay/lesbian community is actively fighting for straight people no longer want. During the past 40 years, the number of divorces has actually decreased, although only because the marriage rate has declined (*Los Angeles Times* 2012). Author and educator Stephanie Coontz claims that married households fell to 51 percent of all U.S. households between 2009 and 2010. She says that marriage is declining because parents today instruct their children to wait to marry until they finish their education and are more economically secure. Much to everyone's surprise, the younger generations have followed that advice and seem to feel less need or desire to marry.

Middle-aged men and women and baby boomers are now dealing with divorce and having to face the dating world. They marry, they divorce, and they marry again. It is not uncommon these days to see second, third, and even more marriages, resulting in complexities and conflict in blended families (e.g., *The reason I divorced my second husband is because I have two daughters and he has two sons. He gave more privileges to his sons than to my daughters. I felt this was very unfair*).

THE AFTERMATH OF DIVORCE

There are a significant number of men who come out of the divorce courts feeling that they have been raked over the coals in alimony and child custody cases by exes who feel entitled to the universe. My clinical, personal, and professional experience has included treating many men who are devastated by their past relationships and marriage, and feel hurt, abused, misused, and jaded about women. They no longer see the need for commitment. They feel emotionally drained and suffocated by court battles involving alimony, custody, unpaid debts. Some men have had horrific custody/alimony disputes, and have faced false accusations such as molestation, addictions, affairs, etc. (While this kind of "court abuse" also can hold true for women, it's been my experience that even though they feel just as jaded, the majority of these women still retain the desire to commit.) For the disappearing male, these influences can exacerbate existing fears centering around intimacy. It is a clinical challenge for therapists to treat these men. Their desire for space, independence, success, sex, and excitement has become a more pervasive force than their desire to forge and maintain an intimate connection.

Renowned author and divorce expert Judith Wallerstein (2000) did an extensive follow-up study on 131 children of divorce. Her findings were that these children often experience failed love affairs and difficulties parenting their own children. She claims they lack the internal structure that models a successful, loving relationship and develop behavior that limits their potential. Children of divorce grow up fearful of relationships and worry that they will fail like their parents. Wallerstein sheds light on the question of whether it is better to stay married and suffer, or to divorce and have children grow up in a broken home environment.

The latter scenario brings up the most common form of disappearing male, all too well known in court systems and custody cases—the absent father who disappears suddenly and feels no responsibility to pay child support or to offer emotional support to his children. In addition to children who suffer the aftermath of divorce, there are children who are products of the effects of war and trauma, as well as latchkey kids—the often isolated and lonely children of working parents. In the past 30 years, there has been a 10 percent increase in single parent households in the United States.

The absent father syndrome has risen in tandem with the escalating divorce rates. In 90 percent of families in which divorce has occurred, the children remain with the mother. While the reverse does sometimes occur, it is more common for the woman to be the nurturer and to care for the children, especially during the early years. The court system has been overwhelmed with child custody cases. The biggest dilemma has been so-called "deadbeat dads." Many women have accused their ex-husbands of maintaining high standards of living while they and their children barely get by. President Bill Clinton has urged the fathers of this country to love and care for their children, and has reminded them that they have an obligation to pay child support after separation or divorce. However, according to the U.S. Census Bureau, half of divorced fathers do not pay the child support they owe. After divorce, women suffer on average a 73 percent decline in standard of living while men's standard of living is increased by 42 percent. Of course these statistics vary from state to state. One study notes that 38 percent of Illinois "obligor" parents not paying child support said they lacked the money to pay. Furthermore, 23 percent used nonpayment to protest a lack of visitation rights, 69 percent complained that they had no say in the spending of their child support money, while 13 percent said they wanted nothing to do with their child or children, and 12 percent denied parentage (Vitz 2010).

Rosalind Zuckerman, a well-known family attorney, claims that a majority of men do not "abandon" their kids. For over 30 years men often have been stereotyped as deadbeat dads, but more recently she claims they have been "reborn." Some men have begun to spend more time with their children for financial reasons: the more time they spend with their kids, the less child support they pay (according to the DissoMaster computer program, which calculates California child and spousal support). Also, Zuckerman's findings show that in many instances the dad is the more nurturing, primary parent while mom is the main breadwinner or a trust fund baby. She also points out that "the way the welfare system is set up, if there is an able bodied man in the home, mom can't collect support" (personal communication, 2011).

However, even fathers who do pay child support can be regarded as abandoning their children if they become emotionally neglectful and unavailable fathers. This can happen if they get remarried, start a new family, and have to deal with the jealousy of the new wife and stepkids. Or they just may have too much shame to face the children they have given birth to and disappointed. Some of these men are what I refer to as "baby husbands," or "baby fathers," men who have not achieved mastery over oedipal issues and remain "little boys" who do not know how to be a father. In one instance, the wife complained that the only way her husband knew how to be a father was to sit on the floor, act like a clown, joke around, or tickle them.

It is also often the case that children who have been traumatized and become victims of unavailable or abusive caretakers end up with severe difficulties with intimacy and commitment. Some female patients have reported having to deal with jealous stepmothers who cannot stand the thought of their man giving money, love, time, and attention to a former wife and biological children and not enough to her own children. In some cases the new wife browbeats or bamboozles the dad into becoming a deadbeat. Child mediators, counselors, and judges alike recognize that when fathers refuse to pay child support they are not only letting down their children, but their families, themselves, and the basic welfare of the society around them.

SUMMARY

This chapter offers a general overview of the disappearing male, taking into account both societal and cultural influences. In the broad sense the disappearing male can be described as someone who falls in love, then quickly vanishes without any forewarning, or as someone who is physically present but emotionally unavailable. While this chapter has provided the groundwork for examining DMS, it has just scratched the surface. The following chapters delineate the most prevalent types of disappearing males—and even take a look at the disappearing female. In addition, they explore the corresponding defense mechanisms associated with withdrawal and isolation in each type of personality.

But first let us turn to the theoretical perspectives that help us understand the disappearing males we will encounter.

Chapter Two

Theoretical Frameworks Pertinent to the Disappearing Male

Although the classical and contemporary frameworks outlined in this chapter embody different approaches, they all share the ultimate goal: to promote healthier intimate relations that enhance psychological well-being. Talk of intimacy must also refer to the defense mechanisms that obstruct it. These mechanisms shape the early way we learn to behave and react to conflict, shield our psyches, and engage with and relate to the world. Today we have substitutes for attachments to intimate objects: computers, iPhones, televisions, social networks, online connections, and other surrogates.

An increasing number of individuals seeking mental health treatment are baffled and confused by a certain segment of people who behave one way at the onset and then suddenly shift to "being another person." Intimacy in this book is characterized in relation to its withdrawal or disappearance, both physically and emotionally. One may disappear emotionally without ever leaving the premises: *My husband is aloof, cold, indifferent, and zombie-like, but at least he is always here* (see chapter 6, what I refer to as The Robotic Male). The perspective of the theorists in this chapter has relevance to the concepts of withdrawal and disappearance that are the hallmarks of the disappearing male syndrome.

CLASSICAL APPROACHES

Sigmund Freud

Sigmund Freud (1923) did not specifically discuss intimacy; his entire focus was on the intrapsychic, not the interpersonal. The interpersonal was intimated by his daughter, Anna Freud, who construed ten different mechanisms of defense and their implication to the ego. Freud previewed the realm of the interpersonal when he discovered transference—the relationship between patient and the analyst. He also proposed the Oedipus complex, which attaches the male child's love for the same-sex parent to the feelings of the opposite sex, a psychodrama of sexual desire for the mother and feelings of anger and revenge toward the father (although if this isn't "interpersonal," then what is?). Essentially, it puts the boy in an uncompromising competitive position of envy, anger, revenge, and rivalry for the mother's affection. According to Freud, if conflict ensues and the child never masters the Oedipus complex, this leads to endless battles and competition with one's mate. One does not have to be a master clinician to figure out how these battles can lead to one partner storming out because of not getting his/her own way.

On the other hand, Freud states that successful resolution of this complex leads one to eventually give up competing with the oedipal rival and moving towards Eros, defined as the desire for love and intimacy. In this case a love partner, a spouse, and a family member may live happily and peacefully side-by-side in a harmonious love relationship. A Freudian analyst relating to a patient suddenly fleeing from his wife might respond with something like: *No wonder you fled abruptly from your relationship. You have not overcome your rivalry with your father. You went against his morality and responded to your impulses (your id). It is hard to compete with a father who is happily married when you are not ready to step into his shoes.*

Melanie Klein

I must pay special homage to one of our masters, Melanie Klein, for without her I would not have been able to understand the encounters that occur among couples, mainly narcissistic/borderline couples (1975, 2001, 1992, 2010a, 2010b). This has specific relevance to the topic of the disappearing male, because frequently it is the borderline that gets "dumped" by the narcissist. Nor would have I understood the introjective/projective process—how one partner (often the narcissist) projects some unwanted part of himself or herself into another (often the borderline), who will identify or over-identify with the projected negativity: *Now you want me to feel like I don't have needs like you, Mr. Narcissist, so now I am a nothing, the needy one, and you are perfect.* I extend this notion to what I refer to as dual projective identification (Lachkar 2008a, 2008b, 2010), which I found valuable in treating couples.

Melanie Klein (1975) abstracted Freud's idea regarding mastery over the father and introduced the importance of the mother in transferring the love object away from the father to the breast. Klein broke new ground with her pioneering work on object relations and her contribution of such defenses as splitting, projection, and projective identification. Her concept of splitting of good and bad objects is known throughout the literature as the *good and bad breast*. Klein believes the primary experience with the breast shapes how the child will perceive the world. If the infant has a good-breast mother, then the infant will grow up seeing the world as good. If the infant grows up with a bad-breast mother, the infant will see the world as all bad.

One of Klein's most valuable ideas was to expand Freud's defense of projection and conceive projective identification as a two-way process. In addition to these formations, she introduces us to two positions: (1) the paranoid-schizoid position and (2) the depressive position. The first position is the earliest state of mind, where primitive defenses dominate. The latter is a whole, integrated position in which one takes responsibility for one's own wrongdoings; works to diminish envy, shame, blame, attack, revenge, magical thinking; and desires to repair and make reparation for the damage that has been done. In the paranoid-schizoid position, the Kleinian therapist treating a patient who is struggling with intimacy may include such defenses as splitting and projective identification.

What follows are examples of how the therapist can make use of these concepts with the vulnerable woman who identifies/fuses with her partner's negativity. It also reassures the woman that no matter how good she is or no matter how hard she tries she will be seen as the bad-mommy breast. Furthermore, it attests to the notion that while these primitive defenses are operative it is imperative that the therapist emphasize it is not a time to make major decisions.

The Paranoid-Schizoid Position

> Patient: *Everything is her fault. I blame her for everything that goes wrong. She gets me so upset I don't know what to do. Should I stay married or should I divorce her?*
>
> Therapist: *It's hard to know what to do if you are in the blame/shame mode. It is hard to think clearly and be able to make a decision.*

The Depressive Position

> Therapist: *No, you are not depressed. You are dealing with normal states of sadness and taking more responsibility for your actions. This is a good time where growth and progress occur and where reparations can be made.*
>
> Patient: *I was wrong. I realize now I was projecting the inadequate parts of myself, because I felt suffocated and smothered. All I wanted to do was*

split and get the hell out! I realize it's okay for me to feel guilty and that was my issue and not so much hers.

W. R. Fairbairn

The work of W. R. Fairbairn (1940) has significance in understanding how and why people stay in painful, conflictual relationships and remain attached to the bad internal object. Fairbairn extends Klein's good and bad breast theory to the notion that people split not into two parts, the good and bad objects, but into multitudinous objects—the attacking object, the unavailable object, the suffocating object, the abusive object, the rejecting object—and forever remain attached to these painful internal objects. As bad as the pain is, it is familiar and preferable to facing feelings of emptiness, or the black hole. Because pain is linked to the love object, it becomes extremely charged and eroticized—"*traumatic bonding*" (Dutton & Painter 1981; Lachkar 1998a). Such bonding creates ambivalence and confusion because the one who threatens and torments can also be loving and kind.

I find Fairbairn's formulations relevant to the disappearing male syndrome, especially for men seeking the unavailable, tantalizing, tormenting, or exciting object. *Well I just don't feel the same excitement as before. I need a woman who excites me!* This can explain how pain can be linked to the love object. This can be very confusing for the woman whose partner can be loving and kind, then suddenly becomes abusive and unavailable. Such bonding creates ambivalence, especially among women who stay with men who stir up wounds of the past. These women are constantly wondering, "Why do I keep falling for men who are always unavailable, who deprive me and give me nothing?"

A Fairbairnian therapist might respond to these distraught women by saying something like: *It doesn't surprise me that your boyfriend vanished. Do you remember from the beginning he was in search of the unavailable/unattainable woman, and you thought it would be different with you?*

Donald Winnicott

Winnicott (1965) is another prominent figure whose unique ideas and language have enhanced and expanded the diversified field of object relations. His focus, like Klein's, was on the importance of the early "mommy and me" relationship. He introduced us to varying kinds of *mothering experiences*—ranging from the playful/creative mother to the containing mother, the being mother, the doing mother, the rejecting mother, the mother of pain, the holding/environmental/background mother. These experiences affect the infant's capacity to be alone.

Winnicott's concept of the "false self/true self" also makes an important contribution to both individual and conjoint treatment. In couple therapy, his concept of the transitional space and transitional objects provides a new opportunity for partners to move away from states of parasitic dependency to interdependency and wholeness. It is clear from Winnicott's work that if one does not have good-enough mothering, the person cannot function as an adequate partner in intimate relationships. For example, a passive-aggressive person will constantly try to recreate the parent-child dyad by engaging in behaviors that essentially state, "I am the baby and you are the mommy/wife who is to take care of me!"

Winnicott felt that the false self was in constant struggle with the true self, or a self that lurks in the shadows and belies the true self. Thus, he may respond to a woman who is dealing with the disappearing male this way: *Your boyfriend reminds me of a Don Juan. Bernie Madoff, a man who embezzled investors, acted as though he was their best friend; some even saw him as a family member and trusted him completely. Sounds as though your boyfriend had an operating system based on a false self.*

Winnicott's ideas are helpful in understanding how a false self can impair a person's capacity for intimacy. For example, Don Juan types have an exquisitely formed false self. Because they lack a real self, they can insert an imaginary one that operates through seductive charm and charisma (Lachkar 2004b). Since they function on the basis of a false self, their capacity to maintain intimate relationships is impaired, and their partners are often duped when they discover that their charming and elaborate promises go unfulfilled.

A Winnicottian therapist might respond with something like: *This does explain how in the beginning he was the ultimate lover, couldn't keep his hands off you, would go to the moon for you, and suddenly changes into a stranger sleeping beside you. He had an exquisite false self. You are blessed to have discovered his true self early on.*

Heinz Kohut

Kohut is one of the few therapists who actually embraced intimacy by his emphasis on such concepts as mirroring, the need for self-objects, and empathic attunement. His approach included supportive interventions, empathy, validation, and understanding the perceptions of others, which are not distortions or erroneous but perceptions that come from an operating system empowered by a person's subjective experience, or "truth." Kohut makes us aware that people with more severe personality disorders, particularly borderline personalities, are more subject to fragmentation and more susceptible not only to disruption in the therapeutic situation but in relationships as well.

Kohut differed from Kernberg in that he believed in the subjective experience as being the truth, that the patient does not distort or misperceive reality. Kohut's work is the most beautiful, warm, empathic as it invites closeness and intimacy. While it feeds the soul, sometimes therapists confuse empathy with containment. It is important to empathize with the feelings, resistances, and the fears, but not with the aggression. Alongside empathy there must be containment. Kohut's work has applicability not only for therapists but for all professionals, businesspeople, and for cross-cultural couples.

Today people are obsessed with talking about their relationships. In fact they are so busy talking about them, they hardly have the time to have them. The capacity to fall in love is a basic human experience, and when people fall in love it is felt to be magical. We all look for the mysterious power of love. Two people begin their relationship with deep feelings of attraction and longing for each other. But lurking in the shadows is an incontrollable impulse to destroy, threaten, and sabotage—a primitive unconscious interference that disrupts love because of an unruly past or early trauma. Sustaining a love relationship can be a full-time job. Kernberg more than anyone recognizes the complexities as he reminds us of the madness of the couples (1995). He notes that relationships are not simple for they are comprised of many complex and interrelated aspects of love, shame, guilt, envy, jealousy, hatred, aggression, rivalry, control, domination, submission, victimization, perversion, pre-oedipal/oedipal conflicts, as well as many early unresolved infantile conflicts. When we talk about marital conflict, we are talking about a kind of love that goes in the wrong direction, primitive idealization that invades and infects the capacity to maintain a healthy loving relationship (painful love, pathological love, and masochistic love, perverse love—and other forms of bonding with the pain).

Otto Kernberg

Shakespeare's play *Much Ado about Nothing* is a drama about a couple that fights, attacks, and virtually attempts to destroy each other. Yet nothing gets in the way of the love: "Love conquers all." The same holds true for Kernberg. In his *Aggression in Personality Disorders and Perversions* (1992), he not only reminds us of the complexities and intricacies of love relations but explains how unrealistic, idealized attachments lead to a reversal of positive love to negative "love," as a consequence of devaluation and narcissistic withdrawal from the object.

I believe that when dealing with the aftermath of disappearing male syndrome, it is important for the therapist and patient to understand what kind of love relationship was involved. There are many different types of love, including: obsessive love, romantic love, erotic/exciting love, idealized love, unavailable love, rejecting love, lost love, sadomasochistic love, repetitive love, compulsive love, and co-dependent love. Pinpointing the type of love bond involved gives the therapist some tools to work with. This is important in helping the patient acknowledge that what she (or he) felt was "love" was not really love. The relationship was more about compulsion, avoidance, obsession, recapturing lost love. Real love is not conflict free, but it should be free of pain and torture. Kernberg's main premise is that no matter what happens, nothing should get in the way of maintaining a healthy relationship—not sex, money, children, in-laws, friends, or any other external influences. For Kernberg the love relationship is sacrosanct. Kernberg (1992) describes four different types of love relationships: (1) normal, (2) pathological, (3) perverse, and (4) mature.

In normal love what is most important is the relationship. The relationship dominates, and primitive defenses do not destroy, infect, or invade or take over the relationship: *I told my parents they could not come over because we needed some time to ourselves.* A normal love bond is defined as one in which the desire to love and maintain a loving relationship overcomes conflict. It is a safe union in which the partners do not feel threatened or envious of the other person's accomplishments, achievements, or attention given to outside "intrusions" (children, family, work, hobbies). Normal love relations entail an already tamed oedipal complex; the desire to love one's sexual partner takes precedence over the impulse to control, destroy, dominate, or compete. Even though many of these couples appear to have a symbiotic fusion, they can still maintain a sense of separateness and interdependence, and live side by side without having to control, envy, or sabotage the relationship.

I can't believe how wonderful my current husband is. Years have passed. We have two children, we both have careers, and are still very much in love. I am very successful and not the easiest person to get along with, but my husband loves and accepts me for who I am and does not try to dominate me like the other men in my life. No matter what, he listens to me, supports my career, helps with the kids. I am truly blessed that I waited until I found the right one. I am so fortunate to have learned from my dating experience not to get hooked up with unavailable men or men who come on too strong. Some of these men were crazy about me in the beginning, but later on started to withdraw and even obliterate me from their radar screen whenever I would share my success with them. At the time I did not realize they were narcissists and couldn't tolerate when the attention was not solely on them. Other men would put me down for being too demanding, too matericlistic, or a "know-it-all." My husband is not perfect, and I do get upset when I catch him on porno sites, but it does not seem to interfere in any way with our lovemaking or intimacy. Of course we have fights and quarrels and cuss each other out. But underneath it all we love each other and nothing gets in the way.

In contrast, in a pathological love bond internal strivings definitely interfere with the capacity to maintain an intimate, loving connection. In pathological love (part object functioning), conflict and primitive defenses take over and overpower the relationship (part object functioning). The result is a relationship filled with shame, blame, envy, jealousy, control, domination, and oedipal rivalry. Pathological love is love that goes in the wrong direction, implying that people who have been traumatized are like emotional cripples in relationships because they link idealization with eroticism.

In the beginning he was so loving and attentive. He loved the way I looked—my sex appeal, the way I talked, the way I expressed myself. He enjoyed watching other men ogle me and felt proud to show me off in front of his friends and business associates. After a while, he started coming to pick me up for our dates later and later. He began to get very negligent. When I finally had the courage to confront him, he blew up, accusing me of flirting with other men, of being too much of a "Jewish Princess" (even though I'm not Jewish, was not having affairs, or using him for what he could buy me). I was completely bewildered because all the things he valued about me suddenly became devalued. I joined a therapy group, which was a disaster. They all jumped on me for not recognizing how from the beginning he was using me as an object onto which he projected himself. I know they were right, but I was not ready to hear that it was my fault. I feel that even if what the group believed was true, he still had no right to abuse me.

In perverse love the desire is for excitement. A relationship never provides enough excitement to satisfy, and the primary goal is to get more! more! more! With the perverse relationship comes a reversal of dynamics. Excitement is good, and love is bad. The vagina is scary and dangerous; drugs are great! In the search for excitement, the good and the bad in a relationship are reversed.

A patient turns to pornography rather than have sex with his wife. As he withdraws and becomes detached, she gets clingier and clingier. In response, he withdraws even further and turns more to porno and perverse acts. As he turns increasingly inward, she attacks. As she attacks, he finds more justification for his perverse activities. In the end, he feels persecuted by his bizarre sexual fantasies and his need to find more external stimulation. With the search for excitement comes an inordinate amount of shame.

The mature love relationship is goal and task oriented and is whole object functioning. It is very much like the relationship of my immigrant German/Polish parents—somewhat boring but harmonious and steady. Kernberg emphasizes that while there needs to be a certain amount of narcissistic libidinal investment in normal love, it gradually evolves into mature love. He claims that the narcissist often drops out during this transitory period, maintaining a plateau of adolescent-type love. Kernberg defines mature love as having the basic ingredient of commitment: respect for the other person's values, traditions, the community, and other links to the love object. *As long as he was in control things were fine, but as soon as I started to assert myself that is when our relationship hit rock bottom.*

For Kernberg (1975) the ego gets top rating. Reality testing and ego functioning are at the heart of mental health. The ego is the barometer that measures mental health, the ability to think, perceive, and see reality. It is the central operating system that helps separate subjective from objective, that involves the capacity to distinguish between self and other and to assess one's own affect realistically. He helps us see how ego weakness contributes to difficulties with reality testing and how this translates into difficulties in interpersonal relationships. His ideas have particular relevance for gaining insight into the capacity for intimacy as interconnected through representations, ego functioning, reality, and the use of defense mechanisms. Although these defenses are designed to "protect" the person, they do so at the expense of weakening the ego's function (reality testing, judgment, thinking, perception). The greatest culprit is projective identification.

The following shows the differences in how a Kernbergian, Kohutian, and Fairbairnian therapist might respond to the distraught patient who suddenly is "dumped."

Kernberg: *You saw the telltale signs from the beginning but you were in denial (ego dysfunctionality).*

Kohut: *This is not your fault. You are not a trained, highly skilled analyst that could diagnose his fragilities when you met. You had no idea that he would leave because he could not sustain the close bond an intimate relationship requires. You had no idea that he would just stomp off and leave you as he did the others. You don't have a crystal ball to predict the future. Even though you saw the danger signs, you fell in love. So you must not blame yourself.*

Fairbairn: *It doesn't surprise me that your boyfriend mistreats you. There can always be an external "mistreater." But you also have an internal mistreater that mistreats yourself and gets in the way of seeing the danger signs from the onset.*

Margaret Mahler

Recognizing the importance of the early mother–infant bond, we must also give credit to Margaret Mahler and her concept of separation–individuation. For Mahler, Pine, and Bergman (1975), the symbiotic period is the first and most significant developmental phase in the formation of object relations. At its core, Mahler's theory demonstrates that fundamental to the process of developing the capacity for intimacy is a successful separation–individuation process, which achieves secure boundaries between self and object and ensures the development of a separate self and identity. Without this capacity, an individual will be overwhelmed with fears of engulfment and abandonment and, as a result, the urge to flee will be more persistent. One of Mahler's most important contributions, which has not gotten much notoriety, is her "practicing stage." This is one of the most fundamentally helpful concepts when dealing with women who need to go on with their lives but are terrorized to move beyond the relationship in which they felt abandoned. To this the therapist must say, Practice! Practice! Practice!

Wilfred Bion

Of all the theorists, Wilfred Bion (1962), a follower of Melanie Klein, provides the most profound and significant links to intimacy. Unlike Klein, Bion sees projective identification not necessarily as destructive, but as having a fundamental impact on intimate relationships. He describes—and thus transforms—what could sound negative or destructive as a form of undigested words not yet suitable for communication. Bion's conception of projective identification is that it is an "unborn" means of communication, an unmentalized experience that is also referred to as a *proto thought* or a *preconception. Did he really mean what he said? Was he just testing me? Does he really want a divorce or is he telling me he wants to divorce the part of himself that has not accomplished anything in life?* This kind of primitive evacuation puts the partner in a very uncompromising position. "Now I have to be his therapist to try to figure out what he really is trying to communicate!" And indeed the partner does need to assume the role of a temporary "toilet breast," a more containing object. Bion claims that the projector needs a projectee to contain these unmentalized enactments. This is especially significant in intimate relations because the partner tends to disavow or not pick up these subtle covert messages. What follows is an example of the unmentalized experience.

> Therapist: *He kept telling you all along that something in the house "smells" and also that he felt sweltering heat each time he entered your house. It was so hot that he was sweating and burning up. You took it personally as if it was an attack against you. What he was really talking*

about is a part of himself that was out of touch with his own internal "smelly" world—feelings of vulnerability and weakness that made him feel bad and rotten inside. Do you realize that these feelings were unmentalized?

Patient: *No, I'm not a therapist and would not have known that.*

Th: *This is why you are here, to understand that when someone attacks you, it is not always about you!*

For Bion (1962) the biggest offense is to avoid the truth when the patient goes into -K link, which means he avoids knowledge-thinking or engages in "thoughts without a thinker." The other offense is for the analyst to *know* in advance what the patient will say or do, or what he refers to as "memory or desire." What follows is an example of a woman "avoiding" what she knew, or in Bion's terms in -K link (Bion 1962).

I just wrote him a long letter telling him how shocked I am by his cutting me out of his life so abruptly, without an explanation or even a return call. I told him that I don't think anyone has loved him as much as I did. I gave so much of myself, even supported him when he was out of a job. How can someone who depended on me for love and support just disappear? To make matters worse, I ran into him at the car wash, and he was wearing a wedding ring. Much to my shock, he calmly told me he married his old girlfriend, a nurse at his hospital. I felt like such a fool. All the while I had a feeling there was someone else lurking in the shadows. Why didn't I trust myself?

In reverse, Bion's concept of tolerance for not knowing also has applicability for the woman who has been "dumped" and becomes obsessed with having to know why. Paradoxically speaking, in this instance the analyst would help the woman tolerate the "not knowing" by serving as the container.

Essentially everything that is happening with Bion is in the here and now. Every session is "now." It has no history, no future; nothing must be allowed to contaminate the purity of the therapeutic canvas. For Bion the only importance is the unknown, the yet-to-be-discovered. Nothing must be allowed to distract from intuiting that. Memory brought into sessions can bring distortions and the influence of unconscious forces. For Bion there can be no thinking from the past or future, but only from the moment. This is where truth lies.

John Bowlby

Bowlby (1969) focuses on the early relationship with the mother as it relates to intimacy, bonding, and *attachment*, a term he uses to denote the child's tie to the mother. His work shows that a child's emotional attachment is a reflection of a child's ability to form secure relationships based on both intimacy and autonomy. When individuals have the confidence that both intimacy and autonomy are available, they not only are able to tolerate aloneness but can feel longing and urges for the love object. Bowlby stresses the difference between withdrawal and detachment. He claims that withdrawal is healthier than detachment because when one withdraws one also withdraws from one's feelings, needs, and emotions. Children left alone for endless hours or babies crying in their cribs without anyone responding to them eventually become despondent and detach. The child's active protestations gradually cease and the child no longer "cares."

For diagnostic purposes when treating the "abandoned" woman, it is important to note the distinctions between withdrawal and attachment. The detached man was never there in the first place! A distraught woman who was recently dumped by her boyfriend says, "Doesn't he even think about me? Doesn't he miss me? Can he just abruptly end it like that? I can't believe all the intimacy and experiences we had together just vanished in his mind." Maybe Bowlby might respond with a statement something like the following:

> *It was obvious he left the relationship abruptly and did not show any signs of missing you. From the onset he had difficulties in bonding. You even mentioned that he had no close ties to his children and had four different marriages. You were complaining he hardly called you or expressed missing you. For him you were merely a love object.*

CONTEMPORARY APPROACHES

Marsha Linehan

This theory retrospective would not be complete without the inclusion of Marsha Linehan's (1993a, 1993b) innovative work on dialectical behavior therapy (DBT). If Freud were alive today he would be quite surprised to find that the world has turned to short-term cognitive behavioral therapy (CBT), replacing his long-term treatment dedicated to probing the unconscious, transference, overcoming sexual impulses, and dream interpretation. Although many of Linehan's theories are tailored for the treatment of the borderline, I find her methodology also applicable for patients who suffer from intimacy and withdrawal issues. Linehan's work on DBT inspired me to create the language of dialectics, which has proved invaluable in my work with borderline patients (Lachkar 2010). Although I see many psychological equivalents and parallels to psychoanalysis, mainly in the complex works of Wilfred Bion (1961, 1962, 1967, 1977), I find Linehan's concept of dialectics far more palatable.

Dialectic thinking is part of mindfulness skills, which Linehan claims are the tools for balancing acceptance and change, or the validating and invalidating environment that is the linkage to self-soothing and affect regulation. Her techniques distinguish between the "wise mind," the "emotional mind," and the "reasonable mind" (Linehan 1993a, 1993b, p. 42). Linehan incorporates these into Mindlessness, a biosocial theory particularly designed for borderline personality disorder. Mindlessness operates within what she refers to as the "invalidating environment" and illustrates how most borderline individuals lack the capacity to focus and are easily distracted by thoughts and images from the past and the future. It is startling how closely Linehan's work on mentalization aligns itself with Bion's concept of projective identification, links on thinking and memory or desire (1967). This is also closely aligned to what I described in my book *The V-Spot* (2008a)—that when one hits a vulnerable chord the V-spot explodes and all capacity to think goes with it.

Although dialectical behavioral therapy (DBT) integrates transference, it applies a cognitive approach rather than transference-focused psychotherapy. The goal is to teach patients to differentiate emotional states so they do not relate each negative emotion they feel to every negative thing that has ever happened to them. For Bion, dialectic tension occurs within the splitting mechanism of the ego: one side loves, the other side hates—resulting in one side that can think and the other side that destroys the capacity to think. One might say that Linehan's emotional thinker is Bion's "thinker without a thought" (1967). DBT is also closely allied to Kohut's concept of empathy and mirroring of the patient's subjective experience. The idea of accepting the patient's subjective experience to be the truth is similar to Linehan's concept of the "validating environment" vs. the "invalidating environment."

Borderline patients are very taxing on the therapist's capacity for empathy and empathic attunement, and DBT helps preserve not only the morale of the therapist but offers specific tools to organize and regulate the pendulum swings and moods of these difficult patients. DBT involves continuous validation and acceptance of the patient's perception as an important part of the healing process, reassuring the patient that the negative experiences really did happen (abuse, betrayal, punishment). Linehan works with two poles: what the patient feels did happen and what really happened. Many of the women involved with men who "disappear" have borderline or dependent personalities and are victims of gaslighting. *Did this really happen? Did he say he had a date with me and then said I was imagining?* Through a composite of Bion's and Linehan's work, the therapist has an opportunity to help patients trust their minds rather than their emotions, which are often fallacious.

Anthony Bateman and Peter Fonagy (2006) developed the theory of mentalization within the context of an attachment relationship. They claim that patients whose inner lives are chaotic and disorganized have a harder time thinking clearly, or "mentalizing." The theory behind MBT is that we develop the capacity to mentalize within the context of an attachment relationship and in an environment that fosters it. Bateman and Fonagy argue that people with borderline personalities have difficulty in mentalizing, making it particularly hard for them to recognize internal states and motivations, especially in interpersonal and intimate situations. Borderlines have a certain vulnerability about getting into intense relationships and then end up being so overwhelmed emotionally that they cannot think clearly. This fits with the disappearing male syndrome. The disappearing male meets a woman and immediately is smitten but does not have the capacity to think about what it means to be with that woman. When he does "think about the experience" or his thoughts become "mentalized," he flees.

MBT differs from DBT in that the former tackles the conflict through interpretation, by helping the patient explore whether he/she is open to alternative possibilities. I am reminded of the patient who assumed in the transference that I was not interested every time I would turn my head away. I assured her that I was so interested in what she was saying that turning away allowed me to think more effectively. What follows is an example of how an MBT therapist would respond to "acceptance" and how a Kleinian therapist might respond to a husband who wants total intimacy and twenty-four-hour "closeness" with his wife.

> Wife: *I know he loves me. In fact, he is very possessive of me. But what also drives me crazy is that he likes to wear my underwear.*
>
> Husband: *But that doesn't change who I am!*
>
> DBT Therapist (to wife): *We have to accept your husband for who he is and not try to change him.*
>
> Kleinian Therapist: *No, this is not who you are. This is a defense against abandonment and separation. You can't possess her so then you become her by wearing her underwear!*

Integrating these concepts of how the cognitive and the analytic approach can apply, or "do the dance" together, are the following examples of mindlessness/dissociation and the unmentalized experience:

- Yes, of course, there can be a real problem in the fundamental relationship, making you want to run away and quit, but there can also be an internal conflict problem that you cause, how you sabotage yourself every time you are on the brink of intimacy.
- You think you need "space" when what you need is intimacy and closeness.
- *"I can't change; this is who I am!" No this is not who you are. You have become your withholding father. Basically you are a loving, kind, and generous person.*
- *"I need lots of women to excite me." No, you don't needs lots of women to excite you. You need to finish your screenplay.*
- *"This is how I feel!" That is not a feeling; it is a defense to run away every time you feel discomfort.*
- *"This is what I think!" That is not a thought; that is an obsession that repeats itself endlessly in your head and never matures into an actual thought.*

Whether the many variations of a state of mindlessness, disassociation, or unmentalized experience are involved, we can reduce these concepts down to one basic fact: the splitting mechanisms that occur in dialectic thinking. The poet Robert Frost may have stated it best in his poem "The Road Not Taken." The myriad decisions to be made in life can lead to inner conflict and turmoil. This parallels a psychoanalytic divergence. The mind splits into two roads, with accompanying ambivalence. The language of dialectics that I abstracted from Linehan's concept of dialectics addresses the patient's ambivalence and splitting mechanisms and attempts to reconcile these oppositional dynamics.

Linehan relates the example of a patient who refused to work on her workbook manual. While Linehan "accepted" the patient's resistance, she also realized that the patient felt that if she did the work she would improve and no longer be in the group. My approach similarly addresses both sides of the split for the borderline but is wary about "accepting" the patient's defenses. If a patient threatens suicide, I might, on the one hand, acknowledge the real threat and check out any dangers of a suicide attempt. However, I would later move in the analytic direction, delving into how the patient is committing emotional suicide. This is my version of the language of dialectics: physical suicide versus psychological suicide.

A. J. Mahari

It is important to mention again that many of the people involved in the disappearing male syndrome are with borderline partners, are borderline themselves, or at least share some similar borderline defenses and dynamics.

Many of these couples are inclined to attack, blame, shame, find fault, and distrust their reality. *Yes, I saw him kissing another woman, and he said I was imaging things.* Mahari's (2009) approach is about survival for the borderline and the non-borderline's dilemma in the relationship. Before we communicate with a borderline, Mahari suggests that we first understand how the borderline sets him/herself up to re-experience and reenact that which feels familiar, no matter how painful it might be (e.g., betrayal/abandonment). Unlike Bion, who gives up "knowing," Mahari prepares the patient—a preemptive strike to offset the borderline's reaction. However, she is in accord with the other theorists about not getting caught up in the borderline's projective identification. *I feel inadequate; therefore, I shall make you feel inadequate!* Mahari, who in the *Borderline Dance* and *The Non-Borderlines' Dilemma* shares her experience as a survivor of sexual abuse and her recovery from borderline personality disorder, makes one of the few attempts to show the non-borderline partner how to communicate.

There are many other contemporary approaches. For example, the Association for Contextual Behavioral Science's Acceptance and Commitment Therapy (ACT) is a behavioral method based on the idea that psychological rigidity is a root cause of conflict, more so than the patient's pathology. This approach strives to develop more flexibility through acceptance, diffusion, living in the moment, and committed action (Hayes et al. 2012). Other approaches include Imago Therapy, Rational Behavioral Therapy, and Experiential Avoidance, to mention a few.

THE LANGUAGES OF EMPATHOLOGY AND DIALECTICS

Inspired by these various theoretical approaches, I devised the language of empathology and the language of dialectics, both abstracted from the analytic literature to make communication more efficient and user friendly (Lachkar 2008b, 2010). These languages are important because we are not only treating women who have been dumped, we also are educating these patients in how to communicate with their partners. Most of these women are dealing with men who have mental disorders, at least the ones categorized in this book. The old ways of communication—e.g., rational thinking, reasoning, requesting an explanation, logic, resorting to nagging, demanding, yelling, gaslighting, abuse, etc. needed a replacement.

Heinz Kohut's (1971, 1977) theory of self-psychology, with its emphasis on mirroring and empathy, compelled me to choreograph a special language to address the vulnerabilities and sensibilities of eight different kinds of narcissists and the various communication styles and techniques applicable for each type (Lachkar 2008). Kohut's empathy and mirroring are essential therapeutic tools in treating narcissistic personality disorders. Robert Strozier

(2011) expresses his utmost respect for Kohut and his theory of self-psychology, likening him to listening to a new symphony, with Kohut in charge of the conductor's baton. Kohut's pioneering work inspired me to compose a new "piece," transposing his concept of narcissistic injury into the "V-spot" (Lachkar 2008a, 2008b). It also led to my formulating the language of empathology, designed to foster communications with narcissistic patients and for teaching those dealing with the delicacy and fragility of narcissistic partners, mainly narcissistic/borderline couples (1992, 2010a, 2010b, 2011), to communicate more effectively with their partners.

Many therapists, not to mention patients interacting with narcissists, resisted and resented the idea of this "special language," feeling it was manipulative, dishonest, enabling, and exhausting. My response is that it brings results and enhances therapy and relationships. The idea originated in several places, mainly in a Macy's department store when I asked a saleswomen who was walking past me if she could help me. She abruptly said, "Wait your turn. Can't you see I am busy taking care of another customer!" (Which I hadn't.) What the narcissist would have heard is, "Mother is taking care of other babies and doesn't have time for me, her special one!" What the salesperson could have said was, "Why yes, certainly. I will be right with you!" What follows is an example of the language of empathology:

> Therapist (preparing a patient to talk to her narcissistic husband): *Honey, before telling you what I need your help with around the house, I first want to let you know how much I love and appreciate everything you do. You work hard, come home late, tired, exhausted. And I understand how helping me is just an added and stressful burden. But without a little help from you putting the kids to sleep, I just won't be able to give you the love and emotional support you need. So if you can give a little time to me, you will see that I will be able to give it back to you!*
>
> Wife: *What! I have to say all that!!! It's more exhausting than putting the kids to sleep myself!*
>
> Th: *Yes, but if you do not try to connect with your husband in an empathic way that he can relate to, you will end up more exhausted in the long run because he will not listen or he will misinterpret your asking for help as a threat or "put-down" and just withdraw . . . "disappear"!*

In *How to Talk to a Narcissist* (2008b), I emphasize how we as therapists empathize with the patient's vulnerability but not the aggression (e.g., *I understand how you feel like beating your wife, because she does things to enrage you, but you are not allowed to hit her*). What follows is an example of opposing conflictual thoughts.

You want to stay with this man because you love him, yet you know he will never marry you or give you a baby. One part of you knows the reality that you should leave him and find someone who will satisfy this need, and the other part is scared and fearful that you will be alone and never find anyone to meet these needs.

SUMMARY

This chapter encompasses a retrospective of both classical and contemporary theoretical perspectives that have influenced concepts and treatment involving the Disappearing Male Syndrome. The theories examined include psychoanalysis, ego psychology, object relations (including projection and introjection), self-psychology, attachment theory, and behavioral/cognitive therapy. The oppositional forces that must be dealt with are: the conscious vs. unconscious; good breast vs. bad breast; knowing vs. not knowing (alpha and beta elements); emotion mind vs. logical mind; the validating vs. invalidating environment; needs vs. withdrawal/splitting/disassociation; success/separation vs. abandonment; old baggage vs. current reality; to think or not to think; to know or not to know; to give or to withhold; to take responsibility or to blame.

These concepts provide a solid base for formulating a sound therapeutic approach to issues centering around intimacy and the defense mechanisms that accompany these issues. I have been particularly inspired by the works of Bion, Klein, Kohut, Winnicott, and Linehan on which I built the Language of Dialectics, which addresses the patient's ambivalence and splitting mechanisms, and the Language of Empathology, which is most effective in mirroring the conflicts and the difficulty in adaptation.

Chapter Three

The Disappearing Narcissist

Wife: *I want to go to the movies.*

Husband: *What for?*

W: *I don't know why. I just want to go to the movies.*

H: *Don't you realize all movies are terrible?*

W: *That's your opinion. It is not my opinion.*

H: *Well, I'm a movie producer. Don't you think I know about the crap out there?*

W: *It doesn't matter. I want to go to the movies.*

H: *So you are devaluing my opinion? I am telling you all movies today suck.*

W: *What about your movies?*

H: *Those are different. They are done with style and artistry.*

W: *So you are the only one who can produce a good movie?*

H: *Trust me. There aren't any good movies any more.*

W: *So your taste in movies becomes the barometer of how movies are measured?*

H: *Look, if you want to go to a movie, then go. I'll stay home and watch sports.*

One does not have to be a psychoanalyst to note the characteristics of a narcissist. Most of us sense we are in the presence of a narcissist because all they do is talk about themselves. The narcissist is the entitlement lover, the special child of God ("His Majesty the Narcissist"). They have a grandiose and exaggerated sense of self, believe the world owes them something and that it revolves around them. They are in constant need of attention, have excessive entitlement fantasies and an overly exaggerated sense of importance, and always demand priority treatment. When injured, they will withdraw or isolate themselves, which often can escalate into narcissistic rage. Narcissists cannot tolerate criticism or take responsibility for their actions and often find excuses to blame others when things do not go their way. When their demands are not met or narcissistic supplies are no longer fueled, they will withdraw or isolate themselves for endless periods. On the surface they appear to have higher than average self-esteem, but, paradoxically, the narcissist's self-esteem is essentially low, and they are quite fragile.

Because narcissists cannot allow themselves the kind of mutual dependency an intimate partner yearns for, they unwittingly project their needy selves into the other (typically a borderline). Not only are narcissists quick to "disappear" from a personal relationship, they are the first ones to flee from treatment when they feel they are not properly appreciated, mirrored, or understood (also known as empathic failure). *It is you that is the needy one! Me, I am as perfect as mother wants me to be! I don't need you, and I don't need this treatment* (Lachkar 2008a, 2008b, 2011).

Narcissists are characterized by a lack of empathy. They are oblivious to the needs, sensitivity, feelings and preferences of others. They value such things as fame, physical beauty, wealth, material possessions, and power. Typically, they were mother's special child until their kingdom was usurped by another sibling. This is known as the original archaic injury. The narcissist is then predestined to spend the rest of his life living a kind of "narcissistic nostalgia," yearning to go back to the time when mommy and baby were one in total symbiotic, harmonious bliss. I often think of my mother, a German/Jewish/Polish immigrant and survivor of the Holocaust, who felt entitled to cut into lines at grocery stores because she felt she had earned "special rights."

FREUD'S VIEW OF NARCISSISM

Freud (1914/1957) was one of the first who conceived narcissism as the state of self-directed libido. The word is derived from Narcissus, the Greek youth of legend who fell in love with himself. Freud viewed primary narcissism as an absolute state in which all libidinal energy is stored up until the ego begins to latch onto other objects and is transformed from a narcissistic libido into an object libido (Lachkar 2004b). These ideas are the forerunners of the notion of self that is between the ego relationship and its ego ideal.

Many women involved with narcissistic men are puzzled as to why they appear so loving, passionate, and available at the onset of the relationship and suddenly turn cold and aloof or just "disappear." Freud explains that in the initial state of love, there is an overflow of ego libido to the object. That love is like a psychotic state, a reunion between highly charged emotional and physical experiences. It is the fulfillment of infantile conditions of love, and whatever gratifies this condition becomes idealized. Passion and erotic desires coincide with the ego ideal. For the narcissist this is only a momentary state of narcissistic nirvana, short lived because of the split between idealized love and the realistic expectations of love. This is the time when the narcissist disappears!

Freud, however, only went so far and did not elucidate what happens to the narcissist when narcissistically injured. Kohut, more than anyone, understands the importance of empathic attunement with a narcissist and how empathic failure occurs. I recall an incident of referring an aging actress to an internist. She went into a complete narcissistic rage after her initial contact with him when she asked if he had all the information needed. He responded, "Oh, yes I have all your information, including your birth date!" This was very insensitive on the part of the internist, and one can imagine the reaction he received from this aging narcissistic actress. Incidences such as this one make me more aware of the special communication narcissists require, for they are the ones who will quickly flee when not appreciated, properly mirrored, or when their excessive demands are not met (changing appointment times, asking for special favors, coming in only when it suits them). Both partners of narcissists and therapists find themselves walking on eggshells, treading lightly and being ever so careful not to trespass into the narcissist's grandiose self too soon.

In terms of intimacy, it is important to note that the way a pathological narcissist withdraws or disappears is quite different than how an obsessive–compulsive or a depressive narcissist disappears. Even though there is considerable overlap, each narcissist has his/her own unique method of withdrawing and putting up defenses against love and intimacy. In other words, each type of narcissist has his/her own V-spot.

NARCISSISTS OFTEN CHOOSE BORDERLINE PARTNERS

In narcissistic/borderline couples (Lachkar 1992, 2004b, 2008a, 2008b, 2011), the narcissist often gets seduced by the borderline's exquisite false self. The borderline play-acts the perfect mirroring object for the narcissist, but the borderline's defective ego and lack of impulse control make it impossible to continue this pretense. The borderline almost inherently knows how to constantly fuel and refuel the narcissist's endless need for gratification and adulation. However, when the narcissist does not pay attention to the borderline's needs or disavows them, tension escalates and turns into retaliation, revenge, and uncontrollable rage that is turned inward. *I dare not criticize him, confront him, or tell him he is not as great as he thinks he is, or tell him what other people really think about him. If I do he'll just take off! Disappear! So I end up doing and saying anything to appease him so he won't leave me.*

The case that follows illustrates this kind of withdrawal and how it is precipitated when the V-spot is stirred and unleashes many unresolved demons in the past of the borderline partner, who already has a thwarted sense of self (Lachkar 2008a, 2008b, 2011).

The Case of Kelly and the Plastic Surgeon

Patient: *When he called and asked me out, I felt as though I had won some kind of an award. What would such a perfect, intelligent, successful man see in someone like me? I know I'm attractive, smart, intelligent, but no way can I live up to his expectations and standards. He's handsome, has a wonderful career, dresses like a dream, has beautifully manicured fingernails, is fine mannered, a physician—my mother's dream. During the entire courtship I felt I never could live up to his expectations. I worried about my hair, my dress, the way I drive, the food I cooked for him. I knew he was a narcissist, but I liked him anyway.*

Th: *Isn't this the same thing that happened in his last two marriages. Bill, your boyfriend, reminds me of your ex-husband.*

P: *My ex was OCD, not a narcissist.*

Th: *There are similarities.*

P: *He would wash his hands a thousand times a day; his food had to be on separate plates to ensure nothing would touch.*

Th: *So your ex feared contamination, that your emotions would infect or make dirt, whereas Bill seeks perfection and cannot allow himself to have needs.*

P: *Why are you bringing up my ex?*

Th: *Because I am struck by how both men make you work so hard to please them.*

P: *You mean what I have to do to try to earn their love?*

Th: *Exactly.*

P: *This is what it was like with my father. I never could please him. Nothing I did was good enough.*

Th: *Is that why you left home when you were sixteen?*

P: *Yes, I had to run away from him. He was too domineering.*

Th: *But you really haven't run away from him.*

P: *What do you mean?*

Th: *You pursue men who are a mirror image of your father, men you can never please.*

P: *So I keep repeating the same experience of hurt and disappointment. Anyway, my boyfriend took me on this lavish trip to Hawaii. It was so romantic. He was like a different person, maybe because he didn't have all the pressure from his patients, the surgeries, the early hours, the midnight calls. It was truly paradise. After we got home I did not get a call from him. I texted him to tell him how much I loved and appreciated the trip, his generosity, and the closeness I felt.*

Th: *And then?*

P: *Still no answer. I started to frantically call him, until my friend said if I called one more time she would lock me in the closet. I waited and waited. Finally he texted me and said he had the opposite reaction, was very disappointed that I had used him and did not once offer to pay my share of the dinners, hotel bill, and travel expenses.*

Th: *That is a shock, especially when he never discussed this in advance with you and because he knows you are not in the same financial position as he is.*

P: *Exactly. This is his problem. He never expressed emotions or what he needed from me, and then suddenly he cut me off. It was always like that. If I confronted him, he just withdrew and I didn't hear from him for days.*

Th: *Isn't this the same thing that happened in his last two marriages?*

P: *You're right! I forgot about that. He would always placate his wife and say, "Fine. Whatever you want to do is fine with me." And then suddenly he cut her off because he felt "used."*

Th: *You mentioned at the beginning you knew he was a narcissist, and yet you didn't prepare yourself for the danger signs, did you?*

P: *Are you blaming me?*

Th: *No, not at all. In fact, I think you are telling us that he is the "plastic man," artificial, not real. But you are not alone. Many women fall for these narcissistic men and are so taken with them that they don't recognize the danger signs. Maybe this can be helpful to you in your future relations. But not if you choose men like your father.*

P: *Plastic man!! Hmm. That is interesting. Didn't think of that! No, I've had it. Never again!*

Th: *Good! Glad to hear it. See you next week.*

Discussion

This patient, like many other women we see today, was highly sophisticated and well read. In fact, many of these women could be writing the new DSM-IV themselves. No matter how intelligent or high functioning, any woman can get sucked in by the charms and allure of the narcissist. In *The Many Faces of Abuse: The Emotional Abuse of High-Functioning Women* (Lachkar 1998b), I describe one of the main differences between the high-functioning woman and the lower functioning woman. The former feels she is not deserving of abuse, and although she is aware of the mistreatment she stays in the relationship for secondary gains (children, family, community). The latter feels she deserves the abuse, brings into the abusive relationship the demons of the past, and bonds with the pain.

Kelly obviously fits into the latter category of the lower functioning woman. She is bright, well read, and well informed, but allows her emotions to consume and control her. This is the kind of woman who bonds with the pain, not because she's mentally deranged but because the scenario is familiar to her. Unconsciously, Kelly repeats the same pattern with men again and again. She falls for the unavailable man, and then wonders why he disappears. In treatment, the therapist bonds with Kelly, is warm, empathic, and mirrors her experience. The therapist shows compassion for Kelly's being dumped, and when the time is right introduces her to her bad internal object (the plastic part of herself). In this case it is the domineering father. Here the therapist plays a dual role, speaking to Kelly in the language of empathology while also confronting her about her dynamics, using the language of dialectics. Part of Kelly longs for a loving relationship, while the other parts try to work through her unresolved issues with her father. It is important for the therapist to mirror back Kelly's experience while at the same time allowing her to heal, to feel and to recognize that neither she nor any woman deserves this kind of treatment.

Now let's turn to the scenario of the married man and single woman. The case below illustrates Richard Tuch's description of the married man, an illustration of the narcissist's sense of being entitled to have two women pander to him, and how he disappears when suitable for him at the expense of his lover.

THE DISAPPEARING NARCISSIST AND THE MARRIED MAN

Richard Tuch's book *The Single Woman and the Married Man Syndrome*(2000) artfully captures the complexities and dynamics of women patients grappling with their involvement with men who are having extramarital affairs. He offers an in-depth approach to this specific relationship and the entanglements the married man and single woman weave while trying to maintain their parallel lives. This detailed portrayal, written by a respected and renowned psychoanalyst, offers a deep understanding of narcissistic men who claim psychological bondage from single women. Tuch does not specifically indicate withdrawal or "disappearance" as a main component of the pain the single woman experiences, but it is essentially intimated throughout the volume. He offers an even broader discussion of women's unique tendency to employ masochistic adaptations in their relations with the two types of men on which he focuses.

The first is the Don Juan type, who wants to conquer women in order to dominate and control them. The second is the narcissistic man who seeks other women to fulfill and replenish his emotional narcissistic bank of self-gratification and admiration. Both these men use and manipulate women for their own self-serving purposes and have their own variation on withdrawal. The narcissistic man will promise marriage to keep the woman on hold—with no concern for her time, emotional investment, or commitment. He will show remorse for not being able to be with her on holidays like Thanksgiving, Christmas, and Valentine's Day and will offer every excuse possible: "Oh I have to be with the family; we have a wedding to attend; my wife is getting suspicious, and I have to assuage her anxiety." Tuch writes with compassion and empathy for the woman who is caught in this bind and is bonded to a man who promises the world and then suddenly vanishes. He achieves his narcissistic indulgence by having not only one woman desirous of him, but two or even more women pining over him (*Look at all the mommies I have now making me into the special child*). On the other hand, the single woman will only have a fraction of a man.

Although Tuch's book does not zero in on the woman's unconscious participation in the abuse by allowing the narcissist to attack her most sensitive area of emotional vulnerability, it does make the point that women get seduced and allured by these painful pathological love bonds. What follows are typical comments from some of my female patients who have been psychologically wounded and emotionally bruised by falling into a relationship with a married man. What these women have in common besides being sucked into pathological love bonds is that they were devalued and abused as children and grew up with men who were abusive or unavailable.

I didn't know he was married until New Year's Eve came up, and he said that he "had other plans." Even though I suspected it all along, it was then I knew. My friend said that when I found out he was married I should have dumped him right then and there, but I always had the dream he would leave his wife. I am now older and still single.

I lost everything. I killed myself for him, did everything for him, sympathized about his pathetic dependent wife and what he had to put up with. He claims he never loved her. And I end up with nothing! Never again! He was just about ready to divorce her when she got terminally ill. He asked me if I expected him to leave her at a time like this. I realized then it was never the time. He remained married and I lonely.

My husband's "lover" called me to tell me what a louse my husband is, that she has been screwing him for over a year, that he promised to marry her, but then realized he couldn't leave me and the children. She said she felt I needed to know what a liar and a cheater he was.

The disappearing narcissist described in Tuch's book clings to an ideal image and seeks perfection in all areas of his life. These men are cold, aloof, often indifferent, and only come to life when in the presence of someone who can fuel their narcissistic needs. When their ideal image is tarnished and they feel sexually and emotionally depleted, they will cut off, detach. They show little or no empathy and feel they do not have to explain themselves to the defeated partner. These are the men who continue on the journey seeking but never attaining an object. Kohut (1977) refers to this as the search for new narcissistic supplies, or self-mirroring objects.

The following cases illustrate how the narcissist feels entitled to exploit women because he sees them as part objects, there to cater to his own self-serving needs, to the detriment of the needs of others: *She gives great blow jobs*. While the men in these cases were not married, the dynamics are remarkably similar to those of the married man–single woman relationship.

The Case of Jan, the Discarded Woman

Jan called up her girlfriend Rachel to report she had finally found the man of her dreams. "Bill is madly in love with me. When we are together he cannot keep his hands off me, and says he has been searching for me his entire life. I keep thinking this must be a dream. After exhausting all the men in Los Angeles and New York, I finally found a man who is totally there for me. He even talks about plans for our future, buying a home, having children, places he wants me to travel to with him. In fact, he sent me a travelogue and asked me to choose any place I would like to visit. What I love about this guy is that he calls me every morning to check on me to see how I slept, how my day is going. And he calls again at night to give me a goodnight kiss."

Meanwhile, lurking in the shadows was a dreamer, full of good-morning greetings and vague plans to travel to museums and castles in Vienna and Prague. Yet when Jan asked when he planned to take her there, he would remain silent. Finally, the response she got was, "I only sent you the travelogue to whet your appetite." Only two weeks later Jan called her girlfriend Rachel again. She was racked with uncontrollable sobs. When Rachel asked what happened, Jan explained how she had been trying to call her boyfriend the entire week to confirm their weekend plans, but to no avail. "We have a date Saturday night, and I have not heard a word back. I am getting very concerned. I call and call and leave messages, but there's no response. Something is wrong." Rachel tried her best to comfort and console Jan, but Jan continued to get increasingly anxious: "I know something is not right; I feel it." When Rachel asked what Jan planned to do, Jan replied, "I am not going to tell you what I am going to do. But I will do it and will call you later."

More calls failed to bring a response. Out of complete desperation, Jane ran over to Bill's office, flew past the secretary, and confronted him: "Okay, where have you been? I have been trying to call you, but you did not return my calls." Much to her shock and dismay, Bill responded, "Please get out of my office. You have no right to intrude here. It's over and finished!" Jan angrily retorted, "Hey, wait a minute. You are the one who intruded. You came into my life with your charm and seduced me into thinking I was the woman of your dreams. Yet, you are not even man enough to return my calls. We did have a date, you know. So what happened? Did I do something to turn you off?" With a cold, austere look, Bill turned to her and said, "You must leave now. I have no time for this kind of intrusive behavior. You are too demanding and far too needy for me. When I did not return your calls, you should have known by my lack of response that it was over."

Cindy, Horsing Around

Cindy was a very successful businesswoman who owned two lovely horses. A fall from one of her horses at a show resulted in a head injury. The neurosurgeon who operated on her fell madly in love with her (and her horses). As Bill did in the above case, Owen proclaimed undying love and particularly enjoyed the gourmet meals Cindy prepared weekly for him on Friday night Shabbat. One Friday she went to several markets as usual and prepared a luscious dinner of roast chicken, potatoes au gratin, and tartetatin. At 6 p.m. Owen had not arrived. At 7 p.m. still no call and no arrival. Out of desperation Cindy began calling him but to no avail. He did not respond to her calls, texts, or emails. Finally at 10 p.m., he answered the phone and abruptly responded, "Why do you keep calling? You know I'm busy and have emergency calls. You just take too much time in my life!" Cindy never heard from Owen again.

Discussion

Jan and Cindy were not physically abused, slammed against walls, slapped, bruised, or otherwise harmed. But the emotional abuse suffered by these high-functioning, educated women can be worse than physical abuse, as many researchers have noted (e.g., Lachkar 1998b). In both cases these women were offered a dream, a delusion. The men knew instinctively how to hook these women, and when they did they suddenly vanished. Nevertheless, there were danger signs that were ignored. The dumped women were so caught up in the dream that they did not recognize the men were "dreamers." In fact, when Jan looked Bill up later online she noted that his profile name was "Dreamer." In the second case, Cindy failed to pay attention to her doctor–boyfriend's violation of professional ethics, dating a patient.

In treatment these women need to know they are not alone and not responsible for the man's sudden departure. The yearning for love and lasting intimacy interfaced with the surface attractions of the disappearing male constitute an irresistible force that can dupe any woman, no matter how intelligent or educated. At the end of each session the therapist needs to remind these women that they have been emotionally abused and offered promises that would never be fulfilled. In future sessions, the therapist can introduce these women to their own internal dreamer, the part of themselves that was stuck in the dream, was unable to see the whole picture, and ignored the red flags.

DIFFERENT KINDS OF NARCISSISTS

There are degrees of narcissism, just as there are many different types of narcissists. Overall, the narcissist is overly self-absorbed and has a strong desire for fame, achievement, and power, to which relationships often play second fiddle. Yet the narcissist still has the capacity to maintain a loving and intimate bond. While all narcissists share excessive entitlement fantasies, it is how these fantasies are played out that determines what "kind" of a narcissist they are. For example, the pathological narcissist feels entitled to dupe and seduce women with a false self. On the other hand, the malignant narcissist feels entitled to turn to sadism and cruelty, while the passive-aggressive feels entitled to use women as caretakers. What follows are delineations of the different types of narcissists that can easily fit into the disappearing male category.

The Pathological Narcissist

The pathological narcissist is completely self-absorbed, exhibiting a delusional, disproportionate sense of self. These narcissists are dominated by such characteristics and defense mechanisms as excessive entitlement, grandiosity, idealization, guilt, shame, envy, control, and domination, which overtake and overpower the capacity to maintain a loving, intimate bond. Their unresolved oedipal issues put them into a continuous state of rivalry with others. Fame, success, power, and constant admiration become more important than life itself. Pathological narcissists are at the high end of the narcissism spectrum. They are totally self-absorbed, aloof, lack empathy, and display total indifference to the emotional needs of others. *I don't care if her biological clock is running; that is not my problem!* If the wife or girlfriend of a pathological narcissist wants to go out for fish, he takes her for pizza. If she wants to go to a concert, he takes her bowling. If his son is in a soccer championship game, he has more important things to do. Pathological narcissists have to be right, and they have to be perfect. They cannot tolerate any criticism, and when hurt or injured will withdraw.

In treatment it is very difficult for pathological narcissists to allow themselves to depend on the therapist, let alone their intimate partners. *This treat-*

ment isn't helping me. My other analyst was far better. To an attitude like this the therapist might reply, "I understand your frustration and how because I'm not perfect like your other therapist you find it difficult to believe I help you. The same thing occurs with your girlfriend; she is never perfect or good enough." Because pathological narcissists show little regard for the needs or feelings of others and have an inflated view that the world centers solely around them, their partners often feel used and abused. *I was at a cocktail party and suddenly he went off without me and completely disappeared.* Typically, the pathological narcissist is like a bloodhound after a rabbit. He chooses someone like a borderline personality type—a caretaker, a victim, who suffers from severe abandonment anxiety: *I stay and keep working on the relationship because I feel that I can fix him!* To this the therapist might retort, "If I couldn't fix him in ten years, how can you do it in a few dates!"

The Malignant Narcissist

The malignant narcissist tends to be cruel, malicious, and sadistic. These narcissists constantly need to have others reinforce their beliefs, traditions, and ideologies. Sadism, paranoia, hatred, and uncontrollable aggression are the most common characteristics of the malignant narcissist, whose self-driving aspirations become the rationale for acting out their worst sadistic and destructive fantasies. The malignant narcissist differs from the malignant borderline in that he has a "conscience" and answers to a higher power. Even though it is a destructive "higher" power, he does have a sadistic superego that kowtows to such figures as Mohammad, Allah, Hitler, Kim Jong Il, the devil.

The malignant narcissist is often a leader, someone who uses his omnipotent sadistic fantasies to live out a cause. Abusive, violent terrorist leaders like Saddam Hussein and Serbian war criminal Slobodan Milosevic may fit this description. Under the guise of fighting for the cause Milosevic killed hundreds of thousands of Albanians. *I swore to the Serbs I would be their protective father and would never allow the Albanians to hurt them again.* These leaders exhibit paranoid and malicious tendencies that compel them to fulfill their self-serving political aspirations and rationalize that it was done for the good of others. For example, Nasser proclaimed that driving the Jews into the Red Sea would lead to pan-Arabism—Arab unity, harmony, and total Arab at-one-ment. Another example is a Muslim man who abuses his wife because under Sharia Law it is acceptable in his country and he must follow the law of his tradition.

Malignant narcissists also find justification in acting out the role of the victim. *We attacked Israel as a defensive operation to defend our poor and homeless Palestinians.* Osama bin Laden claimed the September 11 attacks were in defense of his own people, the "Will of Allah." It is noteworthy that in third world countries the role of victim is a very important part of the culture.

The Antisocial Narcissist

The antisocial narcissist typically presents more serious superego pathology. The antisocial narcissist's most dominant feature is the lack of superego functioning. Unlike the malignant narcissist, the antisocial narcissist does not answer to a higher power, does not have the capacity for guilt or remorse, or the ability to mourn. While, the antisocial narcissist maintains the excessive attitudes of entitlement that are prevalent within the domain of narcissism proper, his sense of entitlement is so excessive that it overrides any capacity for self-reflection.

Two of the antisocial narcissist's most important characteristics are (1) the failure to conform to social, political, moral, and ethical guidelines and (2) manipulative, deceitful, and defiant behavior, with complete disregard for the welfare and well-being of those who are plagued by his focus on his own self-serving interests and desire for personal gain. The antisocial narcissist's most dominant feature is the lack of superego functioning and the capacity for guilt and remorse. Antisocial narcissists may steal, lie, cajole, get caught, and even confess their crimes, yet with no context of guilt, remorse, or concern. Omnipotent and entitlement fantasies are so extreme that antisocial narcissists delude themselves into thinking they can get away with anything.

The Depressive Narcissist

Unlike the antisocial narcissist, the depressive narcissist does have a conscience. However, it happens to be a very severe, persecutory superego that turns against itself. When external narcissistic supplies are exhausted, depressive narcissists sink into a state of morbidity, victimization, and relentless self-flagellation. They are the conductors of self-punishment, and function like a reverse narcissist. Their victimization is a form of entitlement and aggression, a subtle way of coercing others to pity and feel sorry for them. They are narcissistic in that they feel entitled to bring everyone down with them into their morbidity, darkness, and despair about how bleak and empty their lives are.

Depressive narcissists are dominated by guilt and self-hatred. They are perfectionists, and when life does not go their way they blame themselves. They have a sadistic superego that runs amok, and is self-denigrating and self-castigating. Yet, they are highly reliable, dependable, serious, and concerned about work. Their very harsh superego judges themselves as critically as they do others. They are totally self-absorbed and often are withdrawn and isolated from others. A depressed narcissist's grandiose self turns hatred inward to such an extent that it infects and invades all those around him. *I am no longer the handsome hunk I used to be and therefore I am useless!*

The Passive-Aggressive Narcissist

The narcissistic passive-aggressive has an undue sense of entitlement and dependency. He is childlike, irresponsible, and expects others to take care of things while he sleeps, practices the fiddle, and goes to auditions, etc. Unlike the other types of narcissist, passive-aggressives are more about success and fame. Their form of entitlement is about the feeling that the world owes them something and should take care of them. Their passivity evokes rage in others while they do their thing. *I am the baby and you are the mommy/wife who is to take care of me!* The passive-aggressive typically procrastinates until the last minute, feigns inefficiency, and invariably finds a plethora of excuses as to why he has failed to get things done. These narcissists complain that others make unrealistic demands of them, and defend against commitment by forgetfulness, ineptness, and belittling the importance of the task at hand. *I went to the market to get diapers, but the market was closed. I went to get the car fixed, but I couldn't find the keys. I tried to call for a reservation, but I couldn't find the phone number.* These acts invariably evoke an inordinate amount of rage in others. *Now you are the angry one, and I'm just the poor innocent baby husband sleeping on the couch.*

The Obsessive-Compulsive Narcissist

Unlike the pathological narcissist, who cannot allow himself to acknowledge the dependency needs that an intimate relationship requires, the obsessive-compulsive narcissist feels that needs are filthy and disgusting and will spend the rest of his live trying to wipe them away. Obsessive-compulsive narcissists cannot allow themselves to be vulnerable and defend against having needs. They are driven by work ethics and principles. They are also preoccupied with perfectionism and at the mercy of a relentlessly demanding, persecutory superego. They experience the state of dependency and vulnerability as dirty, disgusting, messy things that they project into others. *Don't come near me with your disguising emotions. You are much too needy and all you do is nag.* To offset this, they become obsessed with cleanliness, impulsive cleaning, washing, and a host of other repetitive behaviors. Obsessive-compulsive narcissists attach themselves to objects. They are the collectors, hoarders, and packrats who cannot discard old papers or clutter. Among the most dominant characteristics of obsessive-compulsive narcissists are their anal tendencies, including withholding sex, money, love, and intimacy from their partners.

The Cultural Narcissist

The cultural narcissist will be discussed further in chapter 9. Briefly stated, the cultural narcissist is one who comes into our country waving his nationalistic flag, clinging to the traditions of his birth country and rejecting Western ways of life. The cultural narcissist brings with him a certain amount of nationalistic pride and will hold on to it relentlessly, clinging to his nationalistic or religious identity. These narcissists will not adapt and will do anything to maintain their sense of special identity. They believe that others should conform to their ways and refuse to adapt to the morals, standards, and traditions of our country. For example, *The French are the only ones who know how to cook. The Germans are the best.*

The Narcissist the Artist

The narcissist the artist is in a separate class from other narcissists. Many artists are accused of being "too narcissistic." But are they? When one is talking about creative endeavors, narcissism takes on a different meaning. While clinical narcissism connotes pathology, there are also healthy aspects of narcissism that one might call "aesthetic survival." Clinicians are becoming more aware that the artist needs special treatment, that killing the artist's narcissism is tantamount to killing the artist. The artist needs a certain amount of narcissism to pursue his endeavors. Healthy narcissism allows room for grandiosity, pomposity, self-involvement, and an obsessive investment in perfectionism; yet there is realization of the "need" for the object, the ability to maintain an intimate love bond. There is a sense that the artist requires a transitional space to experience his art. The narcissist the artist is not confined to the performing arts. There are many creative types in the fields of science, medicine, mathematics, physics, architecture, business, and even psychoanalysis who are bonded to their art to the exclusion of all else.

When I first saw her on stage as violin soloist playing the Bach Chaconne, I said to myself that I had to meet this woman. My whole life I wanted to be married to a musician. I took a chance, ran back stage, and much to my surprise she agreed to have dinner with me. Little did I know. We got married, had two children and all I heard all day long were scales and sonatas for upcoming performances. The musical sounds I found so sacred and precious at the beginning suddenly became noise. She did not nurse our children, did not have the time to help them with homework, or go to school events. All she did was practice, practice, practice. I had to become both mother and father to our children. We are now divorced.

Having danced and looked at myself in the practice mirror since the age of seven (what better way to learn about narcissism?) and treated many artists in the Los Angeles area in which I practice has provided me with some in-depth insights into the struggles of contemporary artists. These insights led to my describing "The Narcissist the Artist," outlined in my previous works (Lachkar 2008b, 2011).While they do not all fit into a single category, they all grapple with the same dynamics of shame, guilt, envy, entitlement, and a ruthless need for attention and perfection. Understanding these characteristics is important for therapists who are treating artists (dancers, musicians, writers, actors, designers, creative entrepreneurs, etc.). Therapists need to understand that the artist is unique and requires a special kind of treatment. We must be very careful not to kill the artist's narcissism while we help him/her to embrace the external world and objects.

Destroying the artist's narcissism can also destroy his creative aspirations. For practical purposes, the therapist must understand that even though the person may not be a performing artist, he or she may still have an artistic soul. Therapists must bond with the artist, being careful not to obliterate the grandiose aspects that are essential to his creative endeavors. The challenge facing the therapist is to allow enough room for a certain amount of grandiosity, self-love, and obsessive investment in perfectionism. Artists need a transitional space that allows them to master and perfect their art, but not to the exclusion of others, and especially of their intimate love relations. The therapist must also understand the intense focus of the artistic soul while recognizing how taxing such preoccupation can be for those who must deal with the obsessive focus of the artist.

There is a certain segment of artists who are enormously talented but have a great deal of difficulty allowing themselves the feelings and emotionality required to relate to others—ranging from their love objects to audiences in performing art venues to attendees of business seminars and conferences. Because of their feelings of omnipotence, many of these artistic narcissists lack an internal observing ego and turn to others for constant approval and recognition. Many are high strung, insensitive to the needs of others, and lack the ability to take instruction or criticism. What a bitter paradox: The very things that the narcissist the artist needs to succeed are the very things he or she repudiates: dependency needs, feelings, sensitivity, and empathy.

In writing about, researching, and studying narcissism, and having been around dancers, musicians, and artists my whole life, I can understand how art can consume a person to the point where nothing else in life counts. Psychoanalysis and dance share a mutual desire to express feelings. The dancer uses the body as a vehicle of expression; the psychologist uses counter-transference (or feelings in reaction to the patient). In both fields one has to have enough grandiosity, pomposity, narcissism, and arrogance to pull it off. I'm reminded of the Woody Allen movie *Midnight in Paris*, in which

Owen Wilson goes back into the Golden Era and meets such artists as Hemingway and Steinbeck and confesses that it is really weird for him to be there. The artists respond, "To us that is not weird; we find that perfectly normal. We as artists always live in different worlds."

THE HEALTHY NARCISSIST VS. THE PATHOLOGICAL ARTIST

The healthy artist is always available to learn, grow, and evolve and is able to take other people's advice and critiques without over-personalizing them. In contrast, pathological artists are unable to learn from others; in fact, they often attack or destroy any help they receive that can be beneficial to them. The healthy narcissistic artist is dominated by aesthetic survival, a term I use to describe how the artist remains libidinally cathected to his creative self. Furthermore, they are able to maintain their careers without destroying their object-relational bonds. I am reminded of the famous conductor Gustavo Dudamel, who actually left his orchestra to a substitute conductor to run to the hospital when his wife was giving birth to their first child.

Contrast this with the artists who function at the extreme end of pathological narcissism. They are dominated by such primitive defense mechanisms as envy, control, competition, domination, shame, blame, envy, and self-sacrifice, and obsessed with winning and domination, to the extent of endangering their own health and safety. *I danced a three-act ballet knowing I had torn cartilage in my knee; now I can't ever perform again.* A prototypical example of the pathologic artist is Tonya Harding, who blatantly attacked her rival, 1994 Olympic skating champion Nancy Kerrigan, making it impossible for her to compete in the championship event.

In discussing the differences in the healthy and unhealthy narcissistic artist, what better guide do we have than Melanie Klein's concept of projective identification? In my previous works, I apply this term to couple therapy, how one partner projects a negative feeling into the other, who then identifies or over-identifies with that which is being projected. If we transfer this dynamic to the artist, we can have a better grasp of the distinctions between the healthy artist and the pathological artist. The healthy artist has an outer armor to keep the world from invading or intruding into his creative process. The pathological narcissist does not have this protective layer; rather, he identifies with the negative projections of others and will spend the rest of his life trying to defend against them. The healthy artist does not allow such primitive defenses as envy, jealousy, domination, competition, and oedipal rivalry to infect and intrude into his creative space, whereas the pathological artist does not have the ego strength or impulse control to ward off these external saboteurs. The healthy artist is able to transfer self-love or narcissistic libido to object love or object libido—in other words, to recognize that love objects can actually be a powerful force to encourage creativity rather than distract from it. *When I paint I have the image of my wife in my mind, her beauty, her soul, and her spirit.*

The Borderline Artist

Some of the most creative people have a borderline personality. In spite of their struggles and their chaotic world, borderlines are often extraordinarily creative and successful. One might speculate that because they live within a world of disorder and fantasy, they feel freer and less inhibited. Unlike the narcissistic artist, who feels entitled and special, the borderline artist, rather than feeling entitled, is more invested in shame, blame, and attacking defenses—at his own expense and that of others. There are many unfilled borderline artists hiding in the shadows because of shame and low self-esteem.

Borderline artists have a defective ego and exhibit such defenses as splitting, projection, projective identification, omnipotent denial, and magical thinking. When threatened, the borderline will retaliate, seek revenge, and lash out. Their splitting mechanisms and tendency to find blame keep them trapped in an internal state of victimization. "I give up! I can't go on with rejection after rejection!" This can explain why many borderline artists go into a state of what I refer to as ego dysfunctionality. Lacking the process of the observing ego, they distort and glamorize what they profess to be their real talent. In relationships they frequently disappear, turn to drugs, alcohol, sexual addition, pornography, and suicide ideation to ward off their painful feelings of rejection. Because borderline artists cannot face imperfection, constantly find fault, and look for others to blame, they often play the victimized artist who never gets the same chances that others do.

The Blocked Artist

What is unique about the narcissist the artist is that he has blocked off part of his reality and has made his art the entire focal point of his life. For him nothing else matters, not wife, children, family, friends, or community. His art is everything. There is another cluster of artists who have "disappeared" from reality. The grandiose and omnipotent self has so infected the psyche that the observing ego that monitors the self is virtually nonexistent. These artists believe there is nothing that they can't do and that others will be universally impressed by their efforts. One supervisee came in completely distraught after listening to a recording of her patient's singing, which was so off key that the therapist could not respond when asked, "Well, how did you like it?" She politely said it was very nice, but the patient sensed immediately that the therapist was not blown away by her talent. The patient was so upset with the therapist's bland response that she walked out in a huff and never returned.

Many enormously talented artists have a great deal of difficulty allowing themselves to experience the feelings and emotionality that are required to relate to an audience. An extraordinarily talented and technically accomplished pianist came in for treatment, with a presenting problem involving his inability to succeed in his career. Many of his teachers complained that he was totally devoid of emotion and was unable to express himself. In the treatment that followed it become clear that Mr. X exhibited extreme sexual inhibitions, was unable to free-associate, and had an extraordinarily inhibited fantasy life. He revealed that whenever he would express feelings of emotion as a child and confess his ambitions to his mother she would slap his hands and tell him that he should stop dreaming and grow up. It was surprising to him that as time went on he was encouraged and allowed to express his innermost thoughts and sexual inhibitions. I let him know that his ability to open up in therapy had a direct connection to his musicality and self-expression in his music. As he began to understand how the audience and conductors were the persecutory mother watching over him, ready to slap his hands, he realized how important it was for him to remain increasingly connected with his inner experiences, allowing himself the freedom he never before experienced—an example of the unmentalized experience.

The Victimized Artist

This leads us to the topic of victimization. The victimized artist feels forever frustrated, that he never can catch a break and is faced with a continual stream of rejection and even abuse. Paradoxically, the entertainment world in and of itself is the mother of pain and the land of rejection! It is fascinating that people whose worst fear is rejection will subject themselves to the terrors of auditions and the kinds of humiliation that directors, producers, and agents put them through. Sometimes this can backfire because of the narcissistic artist's lack of observing ego, inability to take instructions from others, and fear of showing emotions.

Therapists should realize that often they are called on to treat the "theatrical" or "musical couple" (teacher–student, choreographer–dancer, director/producer–actor, teacher/conductor–musician, mentor–novice) and the potential abuses that these relationships can encourage. The relationship between teachers and artists is most profound. Not only is it an intimate connection; it requires one never to question but to comply with compete obedience and unwavering submission. If the artist has suffered from trauma or early abuse, he will tend to identify with the destructive aspects of his mentors and teachers and therefore remain forever the victim! The teacher who can be loving and kind can also be cruel and sadistic (a teacher/mentor who abuses his authority). *My ballet master kept telling me I was too heavy, so I lost 15 pounds and became so thin and anorexic that I had to be hospitalized.*

WHERE ART AND PSYCHOANALYSIS MEET

Some of the classical psychoanalysts have addressed the importance of art and creativity and how they interface with clinical practice (Lachkar 2008b). Schopenhauer said that every genius is already a big child, since he looks at the world as a drama and with pure objective interest (Kivy 2011). Freud (1908) searched constantly for secrets of creativity. In his essay *Creative Writers and Day Dreaming*, he asked: "From what source does that strange being draw his material?" He replies that a creative writer behaves like a child at play in that he "creates a world of fantasy which he takes very seriously (and) invests with large amounts of emotion." Freud goes on to say, "as people grow up they cease to play" and that the adult knows that he/she is expected not to go on playing or fantasizing.

I am reminded of a mother I overheard telling her child, "Stop acting silly and grow up!" or "You're acting like a baby." This mother had no clue about Mozart, who was a whimsical, playful, charismatic, game-playing prankster and had a general proclivity for outrageousness. His letters were full of jokes, poetry, rhymes, and wit, reminiscent of one of his most delightful musical compositions, "The Musical Joke." Beethoven is another example of the playful child. Even though Beethoven later became perpetually angry and moody, he had a sense of humor. When one woman requested a lock of his hair, he instead gave her a lock of hair from a goat, which enraged her when she found out.

One of Klein's greatest contributions was her use of the freedom and space to develop a fantasy life in children. She recognized that children have all kinds of sadistic fantasies, accompanies by an inner compulsion to express but not to enact them. This inner violence is an essential element of creative production. Klein noted how the artist can envy others and also be the object of envy. Fear of achieving too much fame and success and thereby evoking envy and sadistic attacks by others can subvert creativity. Think of the film *Amadeus* and how Salieri's envy of Mozart crippled him as a musician.

Some artists cannot tolerate the success and talents of others and will make excuses for their achievements. "No wonder she's a success; she had a mother who pushed her all the way." This is not to undermine the many narcissists, as well as borderlines, who have become enormously successful on their own merits. However, it is important to understand how the demons of their past can sabotage their aspirations as artists. In more severe cases, the borderline artist may struggle and work hard, but if he or she fails then uncontrollable envy becomes the replacement for artistic expression. A good example is the character of Lily in the movie *The Black Swan*. When denied the lead role, she did everything in her power to manipulate and destroy Nina, the dancer who got the part. The narcissist, on the other hand, may be more inclined to make excuses. *Well, she got the part because she was screwing the choreographer!*

Another example is a patient who cannot tolerate any criticism and has an unrealistic belief that he will become a famous rock star. Even after numerous rejections, he cannot relinquish his unrealistic goal. Relatives, friends, and professionals in the field are terrified to tell him that basically he really does not have any talent, that he stutters, forgets his lines, and when he performs is very robotic and unemotional. Yet, he puts the fear of God into them if they attempt to realistically critique his work.

Wilfred Bion (1961, 1962, 1967) offers the concept of containment: if one is going to study and devote oneself to a higher art form, one must be able to handle the feedback and critiques of others.

A young, up and coming dancer enters the class. The teacher, who is French, ridicules the young woman. Most of us thought it was funny, but she was mortified and ran out of class, crying hysterically after the teacher told her: "You look like zee monkey in zee zoo. If you want to dance like zee monkey you should go to zee zoo, but if you want to be zee ballerina, you must look like zee dancer."

Winnicott (1971) in *Play and Reality* noted that the transitional space in which to play and create is essential to human existence. Allowing oneself to play often involves guilt, perfectionism, and an über-critical superego. This is a major issue confronting the therapist. Although Winnicott never studied acting, he had a grasp of the importance of the true and false self, which an actor must be adept at bridging. Joyce McDougall (1995) has devoted much of her career as a psychoanalyst to delving into the mind of the artist and the creative process. She goes so far as to state that even if part of the artistic personality is psychotic, perverse, or psychopathic, as long as it allows the artist to create, it must be considered healthy.

The Case of Stephan

Therapist: *Hi, Stephan. So, what brings you here?*

Stephan: *Well, I am directing a film, and my wife is complaining I do not spend enough time with her or the kids.*

Th: *Oh.*

S: *She is filing for divorce.*

Th: *So, she feels frustrated and neglected because you are devoting your time to the film.*

S: *It's more than that. She started snooping around and found some emails where I was contacting other women who are on the site with me.*

Th: *And?*

S: *She accuses me of having affairs.*

Th: *Any truth to that?*

S: (silent)

Th: *Well, whether or not there is any truth to that, a major complaint holds true—that she feels neglected by you.*

S: *Right!* (feeling relieved the therapist did not push)

Th: *You say you don't have time, yet you found time to contact these other women. So I guess there is more going on than no time.*

S: *You're right. I just don't find her exciting anymore. These other women excite me and keep me going.*

Th: (trying to bond) *You obviously are very creative, and now you're working on your first film. It's interesting that you feel you need more excitement. I would think doing what you are doing is very exciting and challenging.*

S: *Yes, but I run into roadblocks and get very frustrated.*

Th: *Roadblocks!*

S: *The screenplay is much too long, needs a lot of editing, and I know when I confront the screenwriter he will just blow. He does not like anyone to cut his material.*

Th: *So rather than face the screenwriter, you turn to the exciting women to make you feel good and relieve the pressure you are now facing.*

S: *I guess so.*

Th: *Stephan, you are not alone. I understand how sensitive and vulnerable screenwriters can be and how sensitive they are to cutting or editing and take it as a personal injury. I totally understand your dilemma.*

S: *I really want everyone to like me, and most people on the set think I am a nice guy.*

Th: *So needing and wanting approval is very important to you.*

S: (silence)

Th: *Well, maybe I am being presumptuous. But from my experience, most directors and producers are anything but "nice guys" and could care less about getting approval.*

S: *I know. Most of them don't give a shit what anyone thinks of them.*

Th: *That's right. They are very focused and care about one thing and one thing only.*

S: *Yeah, getting it done right.*

Th: *Look, I'm not suggesting you become a real tyrant, but it does sound as though you need to toughen up a bit.*

S: *That's how my father was. He was brutal and abusive.*

Th: *But there is a difference between your father and you. When you confront the screenwriter, you are not being abusive or attacking; you are doing what is best for the film. Your father was just abusive.*

S: *So you're saying I need to have more balls!*

Th: *Ah! Yes! And this is where the real excitement lies, not with a few romances or hits on the Internet. We need to stop now and shall continue on next week.*

Discussion

The therapist was very careful not to confront Stephan about the possible affairs, but to focus more on bonding with the patient and his uncontrollable need for excitement as a split-off defense. Mirroring his difficulty in confronting the screenwriter and showing empathy opened the door to Stephan's V-spot—the need for others to like and approve of him. In this case the therapist avoided talking too much and asking too many questions, thus bombarding Stephan with too many words to process at once. Rather, the therapist listened attentively and allowed the problem to unfold gradually. The thematic material lent itself to an association with an abusive father, Stephan's distorted image about manliness, and his confusing abuse with being a good director.

The therapist then drew on her own experience with directors and producers to let the patient know it is his role to confront the screenwriter (therapist as the containing object) and how this can lead to having "real balls." The therapist also helps Stephan understand that he needs a certain amount of vulnerability and observing ego to pursue his artistic endeavors. The side benefit is that being vulnerable also is a major ingredient for a relationship. ("Yes, it is okay to emote when playing the drums. Practice first with your love partner and these feelings will carry over to your music." My association was with Schumann, who created the most gorgeous music for his wife, Clara, the love of his life!)

THE THERAPIST'S ROLE

Freud in *Moses of Michelangelo* (1914) pointed out that psychoanalysts and artists have one thing in common: their ability to tolerate things in life that are not neatly packaged and harmonious. Every attempt to create order must have an equal amount of disorder. When treating the artist, it is important for the therapist to remain aware that the artist must possess a grandiose self and enough arrogance to pull it off; however, this should not replace feelings and vulnerability. The very nature and culture of the performing arts field is prescripted for narcissistic injuries (rejection, envy, rivalry, betrayal, waiting, competition). The therapist treating the artist must be aware that:

- Envious, destructive teachers, choreographers, conductors, producers, bosses, mentors can stir up archaic injuries stemming from parental neglect and abuse.
- Legitimate issues facing the artist include aging, physical injuries, diminution of mental faculties, loss of talent and beauty.
- The artist needs an outer shield/protective layer in order to take injury, criticism, judgment, corrections, pain, and adversity.
- Dependency needs and feelings of vulnerability are an integral part of the creative process, as well as of love relations.

The relationship between the therapist and the artist should be based on trust. A challenge for the therapist treating the disappearing artist is the maneuvering required by the narcissistic artist's overly exaggerated sense of entitlement. When they are in relationships, they often depend on their partners, family, and friends to support them while they pursue their career. It goes without saying how this can put an undue amount of stress and pressure on relationships, in addition to the stress already experienced by the woman who feels her partner has abandoned his responsibilities.

It is not uncommon for disappearing narcissistic artists to find justification for their overly entitled selves by referring to great painters or composers of the past who expected to have their genius coddled, stroked, and nourished. Society masked their dependency by petting and abetting them. It was prestigious to be known as a patron of the arts. Artists and musicians were recognized for their talent and skill and were supported by kings, popes, and aristocrats. It was acceptable that they could have tantrums and act "crazy" as long as they displayed great genius (e.g., Beethoven, Bach, Mozart, Michelangelo, Leonardo da Vinci). Society became tolerant of the "artistic mood" and even came to expect nonconformist behavior.

However, patronage isn't what is used to be, and the narcissist the artist currently faces fierce competition for recognition of his talents. An artist can no longer afford to believe that "I can't diminish myself or my talent by getting an everyday job." To this way of thinking, the therapist can respond that many artists were bankers, butchers, plumbers and had large families to support. Mussorgsky was in the military, Matisse was a lawyer, Chekov was a doctor, and Borodin, a chemist. Anaïs Nin wrote pornography, Dickens wrote serial articles for newspapers, and Mozart wrote "junk music" for extra money.

Therapeutic bonding with the artist includes acknowledging the importance of the grandiose self and gradually chiseling away the part that infects and invades his object world. To treat the artist effectively, the therapist must:

- Provide a safe environment that allows the artist to express his feelings, emotions, and fantasies and be the playful child.
- Help the artist disidentify with the negative projections commonly stirred up by teachers, bosses, and mentors.
- Be aware that omnipotence is a double-edged sword; it is important for drive and motivation but not for performance, which requires emotion and sensitivity.
- Show the artist how love relations embrace and enhance creativity rather than distract from it.
- Recognize that the artist responds more to mirroring, emphatic attunement, and interpretation as opposed to confrontation.
- Gradually wean the artist away from a self-directed libido toward awareness of outer reality.
- Assist the artist in understanding that criticism is essential to the creative process.

In treatment we must always show respect for the very real losses that artists may be dealing with (injuries, loss of beauty, aging, loss of skill/technique/status in society) and remind them that they should never lose sight of their artistic soul. The artistic soul never dies. Once an artist always an artist. This holds true for artists in any field, even if they are not performing for audiences. Their artistic sensibilities constitute a great part of their identity.

I remember seeing my analyst after a terrible ballet class. I told him that I just hadn't done well that day. He turned and looked at me and said, "Why should that matter? You are not going to be a professional dancer anyway." Somehow when he said that something in me died. I did not dance with the same vigor and vitality.

SUMMARY

The relationship between the therapist and the artist can be a most creative, moving, and rewarding experience. However, we must remember that we are dealing with a specific group of people who are extraordinarily vulnerable and sensitive to the reactions and responses of others. The healthy artist, however, is able to block out the negativity and stay connected to his/her own internal world, whereas the unhealthy artist will readily identify or over-identify with the negative projections of others. Therapists who understand the issues that artists in all types of fields face can provide some valuable tools to help these individuals grow and develop not only in their artistic world, but in a healthy interpersonal one.

Chapter Four

The Disappearing Borderline

We are the Hollow Men. We are the victims. We are the abandoned ones.
We are the lost souls, the empty ones. We will get revenge.
We will get even. You will live through our pain.

DEFINING THE BORDERLINE

Although Freud was not a social psychologist and did not make reference to the term "disappearance," he did include within the mechanism of defense the notion of dissociation. Borderline was not a term on his radar screen. However, he noted early on that there was a certain segment of patients who could not tolerate success. As soon as they neared the pinnacle of success, they would go into a massive regression. They would also sabotage any progress they made in treatment.

Borderlines suffer from severe abandonment anxiety. These are the males who were emotionally abandoned in early life by parents who were absent, alcoholic, abusive, or physically or emotionally unavailable. They frequently perpetuate the cycle by staying in abusive, addictive, or obsessive relationships, enacting the role of victim (bonding through pain either self-inflicted or other inflicted). The most prevalent dynamic is the tendency to overreact to even minor criticism.

Because of a childhood of trauma, abuse, and deprivation, the disappearing male borderline becomes insatiable and demanding—always wanting but never receiving. The borderline is the one with not only a broken heart but a broken ego, a fragmented ego that distorts reality into fantasy and wishful or magical thinking. The borderline has a defective sense of self, emanating from early trauma that affected the maternal attachment bond and resulted in an over-concern with the "other."

The disappearing borderline has a heart that wants to heal but finds avenues that cause the emotional arteries to self-destruct. Unlike the narcissistic, whose major intent is the search for approval and accolades from self-objects, borderlines are desperately seeking bonding. Unfortunately, because of the lack of impulse control, combined with destructive impulses, feelings of persecutory anxiety, and the false self, they cannot maintain an intimate, loving relationship. Instead, they inevitably destroy it. Borderlines suffer from severe abandonment anxiety, do not have a sense of self, do not feel entitled, and do not care about success, fame, power. Instead they are more preoccupied with proving a sense of existence because they felt abandoned in early life.

My mother was often either asleep or medicated. When she was better, she would paint what she thought were great works of art but which were painfully atrocious. Visiting my mother was excruciating agonizing. Her house was a mess, full of old papers, old collectibles. She was a total pack rat. She would sit with her eyes "out to lunch," staring into space. She rarely had contact with others, and the only pleasure she got was from her artwork. I didn't dare tell her how dreadful it was.

Borderlines are the victims, the scapegoats, and when betrayed will spend the rest of their lives getting even, getting back. They will sacrifice themselves, their children, and their families in the quest for revenge. This makes them easy prey for the seductions of someone like a dependent personality or caretaker-type woman who thrives on feeling needed (Lachkar 1992, 1997, 2008b, 2011).

I stay with this man even though he abuses and tortures me. My friends have stopped listening to my complaints. They tell me I am a victim and should go on with my life. They don't understand how terrified I am to be alone. Better to be in a bad relationship than to be alone and feel a sense of nothingness. At least when I am with him, as bad as the pain is I feel alive!

In order not to feel abandoned, borderlines learn how to enact the role of being the perfect mirroring object, especially for a narcissist. *I'll do anything. Just don't abandon me!* But because of their lack of impulse control, their mirroring is short lived. Borderline men are very luring and seductive. They are the Don Juans, the Romeos, the savvy lovers who are adept at pulling the wool over the most discerning eyes. Many women have been hurt and emotionally injured by these borderline men. They operate through an exquisitely formed "false self" (the self that belies the "true self"). In conjoint treatment, even therapists often get sucked in by their unwaveringly irresistible persuasion, their role as victim, and their seductive lures, making it difficult to diagnose these charming men from the onset.

EVER THE VICTIMS

I refer to the brand of seduction that is the hallmark of borderlines as the "Michael Jackson Syndrome." Because of Michael's persuasive pleas about his desperate need to sleep and to perform at his best, his doctor easily was sucked into Michael's demands. The threat that hangs over such powerful borderlines is that if we don't comply, they will act out destructively. They will attack us, get sick, suspend payments, miss appointments, and offer a barrage of reasons why they were late or couldn't make their appointments. We often answer borderlines' out-of-session calls because we are fearful that they are having an emergency. What counts as an emergency to a borderline is more about feeling explosive inside, like an over-heated pressure cooker. What a therapist regards as an emergency is another story. We as caretakers are easily taken in by the borderline's victimization act. Yet, we are not alone. Others fall into the same trap. Borderlines are the ones who tie up the court system. They use pain as a means of getting people to feel sorry for them (psychosomatic illness, addictions, suicidal ideation). *When I burn myself with a cigarette, then I know I'm alive. I exist! Anything is better than abandonment! Drugs, alcohol, even this terrible abusive/addictive relationship! As bad as the pain is, it is still better than having to face the meaninglessness, the abyss!*

Borderline personality disorder is frequently co-diagnosed with other conditions, including bipolar disorder, major depression, anxiety disorders, and substance abuse. It is very easy to confuse bipolar disorder with borderline personality. There is definitely an overlap. Both the borderline and the bipolar have mood swings, and both have difficulty dealing with outbursts of rage and bouts of depression. Both also lack impulse control. The difference is that people with bipolar disorder can function relatively normally between episodes, whereas the borderline lives in a chronic state of chaos and instability. Bipolar depression may linger on for weeks, whereas the borderline may be in a continual state of short-lived episodes of anger, rage, attack, and shame/blame. These are often linked to bouts of impulsive acting out and aggression, self-inflicted injury, abuse, victimization, and addiction—including drugs, alcohol, sexual addiction, and the formation of masochistic or sadomasochistic attachments. *I was functioning fine, felt stable, confident and all of a sudden I felt a tingling in my body, and I knew I was going to have an episode. As hard as I try to control and fight it, I can't.*

Distorted cognition and sense of self in borderlines can lead to frequent changes in long-term goals, career plans, jobs, friendships, gender identity, and values. The term bipolar says it: there are wide mood swings that range from one extreme to the other. When manic, they feel they can conquer the world; when depressed they feel hopeless and nonexistent. Depression, mania, and other mental states are part of the mix. In addition, the bipolar is more inclined to have a chemical imbalance and be in need of medication. To safeguard against misdiagnosis, borderlines need a psychopharmacological work up.

In *How to Talk to a Borderline* (Lachkar 2010), I start by welcoming the reader to "Borderland," a world that knows no bounds and breeds a uniquely complex and fascinating group of individuals. This is not meant to be pejorative in any way. It's just a fact that the borderline's world is not based on reality. They are the most puzzling and difficult-to-treat patients, who can baffle even the most seasoned therapist. Yet, they can also be the most perceptive, insightful, and extraordinarily creative and artistic group. Marsha Linehan (1993a), a foremost expert on borderline personality disorder, notes, "Borderline individuals are the psychological equivalent of third-degree-burn patients. Lacking the emotional skin, they feel agony at the slightest touch or movement."

> Wife: *Why are you just sitting there? Why don't you go out and find a job?*
>
> Husband: *I did find a job. I found three jobs.*
>
> W: *But you got fired from all of them.*
>
> H: *Yes, but you need to understand it was not my fault.*
>
> W: *You are always blaming other people and never take any responsibility for your mistakes.*
>
> H: *Look, this boss was an asshole!*
>
> W: *That's what you said about all the other bosses. Why don't you for once take responsibility? You were always arriving late, wore sloppy clothes, angered your customers.*
>
> H: *Goddamn it! You are always taking the sides of other people and blaming me for everything.*
>
> W: *I blame you because you were wrong and now you don't have a job.*
>
> H: *Fuck you!*

The borderline will self-mutilate, pull hair, overindulge. He lacks impulse control and will do anything to subvert an intimate connection. Domination, control, and victimization are the defenses he uses to guard against weakness and vulnerability. People (including therapists) intuitively understand not to "rock the boat" when in the presence of a borderline. They walk on eggshells because one wrong move or word and the borderline will blow, what I call the "V-spot explosion." Borderlines are very taxing on the therapist's empathy.

I tell her she was late again for her session. She says she is never late. I remind her about last week when she got stuck in traffic. She then responds that it didn't count because it was not her fault. I knew better than to say that I have a record in my notes indicating how many times she was late for sessions. To do so would precipitate an endless battle. I have quickly learned to avoid engaging in battle. Borderlines are like a slippery slope. I never can win!

One patient, a violinist, instructs me to never mention famed violinist Jascha Heifetz. She says that when I do she feels as though she disappears. This may sound narcissistic, but it has borderline overtones. As soon as his name is mentioned, she feels she no longer exists.

Borderlines are always trying to prove their sense of existence as a thing in itself (Lachkar 1992, 1997, 2008). In contrast, narcissists already know they exist and are busy trying to prove their "special sense" of existence. *I am mother's special child.* The narcissist at least knows he exits, whereas the borderline has disappeared from himself. *I only exist when I am in pain, when you are with me and I know you won't leave me.* In addition, unlike the narcissist, borderlines are more impulsive, less stable, more clingy, self-destructive, self-defeating, and bond with others through pain and victimization. The narcissist bonds with the Mother of Entitlement. The borderline, in order to achieve some semblance of existence, bonds with the "The Mother of Pain," the victimized self. *I know I don't have the money, but when I shop I know I am alive! As bad as I feel the next morning at least it is still better than having to face the meaninglessness, the dread, the abyss!*

A great deal of confusion exists about the borderline, but one of the things most therapists agree on is that they must find a hook, a way to bond with them. The following example illustrates the therapist's use of the language of dialectics to address the borderline's boundary confusion. As much as the borderline hates his mother, the therapist shows how he has become her!

Tom was referred by a friend who was the relative of a very well-known movie director. It was intriguing for me to study the types of individuals who come from families with so much fame and wealth yet produce children with

BPD. Even though I knew this patient was going to be quite a challenge, my interest and intrigue overcame my doubts. Tom was exactly the type of man whose pathology prevented him from having a lasting intimate relationship. Because of his blurred boundaries, confusion, and delusions, he lacked the observing ego mechanisms to realistically monitor how his behaviors could be a turn-off not only to women but to others with whom he interacted. Tom disappeared from his reality into a world of blame, shame, and attacking defenses.

At the onset of treatment, Tom was notoriously late for his appointments. However, as treatment progressed he began to show up closer and closer to the appointment time, and in some cases even arrived early. Tom would do fine for a while. However, if I even hinted that there was any kind of defect within him that caused other people to respond to him the way they did, he would go into an uncontrollable rage. *How dare you say that! You are fucked up just like everyone else. My parents did bad things to me, and it is entirely their fault. If it weren't for them, I would have a nice life and wouldn't be sitting here talking to you!* This case illustrates not only identification with the bad-breast mother but, much to Tom's surprise, he learns he actually becomes her.

The Case of Tom

Therapist: *Hi, Tom.*

Tom: *Hi!*

Th: *I see you are a half hour late. That doesn't give us much time.*

T: *That's because my mother's always late.*

Th: *So you blame your parents for your problems?*

T: *Yes, my mother used to throw me against the wall and do all kinds of bad things to me.*

Th: *Then you were abused? Where was your father?*

T: *He did nothing, the asshole.*

Th: *So in a way you are like your mother. When you get angry you become abusive.*

T: *I am not abusive, and don't you dare tell me I am like my mother!*

Th: *You're right. You are not like your mother. Your mother would never go to therapy to get help. At least you are here, and I commend you for that.*

T: *Oh, yeah. I guess that's good.*

Th: *Even the way you get angry is different than your mother.*

T: *Like how?*

Th: *The cops got angry with you for parking in the wrong space last week, but they were doing their job. Your mother got angry with you because she did not do her job. She did not have the parenting skills to discipline her child* (fusion with the "bad, unjust cop mother").

T: *No, she was an idiot who didn't know from nothing.*

Th: *So, basically, when I mentioned the car-parking incident, we were talking about boundary confusion: what you did, what the cops did, and what your mother did. She was your mother, but she didn't act as a mother should. Just as you didn't act like a good driver and park in a space provided for cars* (the language of dialectics).

T: *Wow! This is great. I never thought about this before.*

Th: *I see you have analytic insights, Tom. This can be very helpful to us. I am impressed. We have to stop now. See you next time.*

T: *Why do we have to stop? It was not my fault I was late.*

Th: *But if I continue and my next patient comes, then I would be parking in the wrong space, just like you did with the car. You have your space and I have mine.*

T: *Okay, got it. See you next week.*

Th: *Good work, Tom.*

Within the context of this book, I view the borderline males as eternal little boys. They are the ones who pretend to have daddy's penis; however, developmentally they have not evolved, so they end up play-acting, putting forth the false self. The borderline is similar to the passive-aggressive. The difference is that the passive-aggressive does not express his rageful self overtly. The passive-aggressive covertly coerces his partner to enact out his rage by continuously setting up the child/parent dyad (see chapter 7).

WHAT MAKES A BORDERLINE CHOOSE THE NARCISSIST?

Borderlines often join up with a narcissist. Because borderlines have a defective sense of self and are beset by feelings of nonexistence, unworthiness, lack of entitlement, they are mesmerized and easily seduced by the narcissist's omnipotent and grandiose qualities. *You are the most beautiful woman in the world—the most perfect and the most special.* Borderlines delude themselves into thinking that the narcissist is "everything" and that they are "nothing." They fantasize that the narcissist offers some semblance of power, grandiosity, and entitlement to the split-off needs they have long ago abandoned and still crave. Instead of standing up for these needs, they form parasitic attachments through seduction, manipulation, victimization, and pain. In order not to feel abandoned, borderlines learn to play into their partner's narcissism, and for a short time can enact the role of being the perfect mirroring object. Oftentimes borderlines attach themselves to the "unavailable object." Unlike the narcissist, borderlines do allow themselves to be dependent, but then feel persecuted by their dependency needs and react accordingly.

I am madly in love with a man, but I never know when he is going to show up. He travels a lot, but just when we start to get close he does something to sabotage our relationship. He accuses me of seeing other men, gets crazed with jealousy, looks through my email, and makes a big deal of the slightest suggestion of another man being interested in me. He lacks boundaries and has total disrespect for my privacy. He just shows up at my condo whenever he likes, and when I question him, he gets enraged and accuses me of not wanting him. I always tell him that wanting to know when he is going to show up has nothing to do with not wanting him there. He then distorts and misreads what I say to mean, "Sure, you want me to tell you in advance in case there is another guy at your place." Although I know he will always show up eventually, he is not there for me emotionally. All he does is shows up in the middle of the night so he can get laid.

Miraculously, with the skill of a fox, borderlines often seem to sniff out narcissistic women whom they praise, admire, and adore. Eventually this idealization wears off and the borderline's true self begins to emerge—mainly because of the borderline's lack of impulse control and his inability to contain. Does the love disappear? Was it fake? Many women (and men, of course) ask this question. It can only be answered in general terms. The way the borderline disappears is different than the way their other disordered brethren vanish. The borderline will cajole, manipulate, and betray. Borderlines suffer from privation rather than deprivation, illusions rather than delusions or hallucinations.

BORDERLINE ENVY

In my experience with borderlines within a marital love bond, it is not unusual for the borderline to fall in love with a successful, smart woman, only to find that in time her success becomes his demise. The relationship is what I refer to as the "baby husband and the mommy/wife he must destroy."

I don't understand why he destroys everything good. Whenever I get a bonus or a raise, I would think he'd be happy. Instead, he just frowns and then disappears! He also keeps me so preoccupied wondering what he's going to do and trying to understand the chaos that I can't even concentrate on my work. I spend most of my time checking his emails to see if he is contacting other women or spending time on porno sites. He lies to me, and when I confront him he tells me I'm imagining things. He even sabotages our time with the kids. Doesn't he want us to be happy?

What confuses most women is that no matter how successful, how beautiful, how brilliant, how soft their skin, they can become the target of borderline envy. The borderline's destructive attitude toward his partner has no bounds. *The more I give, the meaner and crueler he is to me.* Because he is threatened and envies her, the borderline must destroy her. Borderlines suffer more from privation than deprivation. They never had the experience of bonding that the narcissist once had. Therefore, instead of allowing a budding relationship to feed and nurture them, they must destroy and sabotage it. The borderline may stay away; suddenly stop calling, texting, and emailing; have affairs; do anything to stir up insecurity and confusion in the woman that is envied. The most common dynamic is revenge. *Now I am the one in control, and she is the helpless victim.* The desire for revenge dangerously increases the aggression, sadism, and chaos, and dramatically changes the love partner into a rival (Kernberg 1975). *Okay, I'm sorry. I will never ask for anything again!*

Romancing the Borderline: The Case of Allison

As I was writing this book, I received a desperate call from a woman living in Ireland who met a British man on a cruise ship. She requested a long-distance therapeutic session with me and started off by asking if I had ever heard of the syndrome of a disappearing man. I wanted to burst out, telling her that was exactly what I was writing about at that very moment. Knowing that I must not contaminate the therapeutic space, as Bion reminds us, I held back at first, waiting to see what would transpire in the session.

Therapist: *Hello, glad you were able get the start time right. It is my morning and your night.*

Allison: *Yes. I was very anxious to talk to you because I read your book* The Narcissistic/Borderline Couple, *and I am convinced that I am the borderline and my past boyfriend a narcissist.*

Th: (listening attentively)

A: *I always felt good about myself, thought of myself as intelligent and attractive. But after I met Walter, I started to doubt myself.*

Th: *How did you meet Walter?*

A: *We met on a cruise ship. Right away he expressed his deep feeling for me, that it was love the moment he set eyes on me. He said for him I was the perfect woman—beautiful, charming, intelligent—and that he had never experienced a throbbing in his heart before like this.*

Th: (listening)

A: *He said he wanted to take me to London to meet his family. He said he would be there for me and even look after me financially if need be.*

Th: *Did it surprise you that he came on so strong?*

A: *Yes, it did. But he was so convincing, and I was feeling so desperate after my last boyfriend, who made me feel like an abject nothing. I was just soaking this in. But I did notice he would get very distant whenever I questioned anything about his past or his past relations. He was always quick to change the subject. Nevertheless, he just showered me with flowers, gifts, and cards, and before I knew it we were having sex.*

Th: *So you did notice some red flags. But because you were desperate and still in mourning over the break-up of your last relationship, you overlooked that he was evasive and dismissive of you and your curiosity.*

A: *Yet he was not curious about me at all. Never asked any questions, never indicated feelings of jealousy if I ever brought up my exes. I am still in love with him, even though I know now he is a womanizer. I read some of the emails on his iPhone. I know it wasn't right, but I couldn't help myself. Then suddenly he just stopped calling me, and I cannot get him out of my head.*

Th: *Allison, this doesn't sound like love. This sounds like an addiction. You have become obsessed with him.*

A: *You're right. I keep wondering, did he really mean it when he said he was taken with me at first sight, or did he make that up? I can't get those words out of my head, and I keep wondering if I'm crazy or if he really meant it.*

Th: *Allison, as you know, I can't analyze someone I have never evaluated, but based on what you said he sounds more borderline than narcissist.*

A: *Borderline? I have read many books on the borderline and never thought about him that way.*

Th: *For our purposes here, let us assume for the moment that he is borderline. What do we know about borderlines?*

A: *From what I have read, they have great deal of difficulty with bonding and attachment.*

Th: *Excellent. Let's take that a step farther. In the beginning, he sees this beautiful woman, becomes smitten, and is overwhelmed with a gush of feelings for her. And then suddenly he disappears.*

A: *Yes, that's what I want to know about.*

Th: *I can't speak for Walter, but what we do know is that borderlines have a great deal of difficulty maintaining object constancy, and when they start to get feelings of love they split off.*

A: I *don't understand how a man so in love can do that—even a borderline.*

Th: *Allison, it would be as if I went to a Rolls Royce showroom, fell in love with a Rolls, and said to myself, "That car is a beauty, and I must have it." Then afterwards I would realize that as wonderful as the car is, how would I keep and maintain it? It would deplete me economically. Walter's desire for you would deplete his emotional resources. He has not yet acquired an emotional bank.*

A: *It makes me feel better that you think of me as a Rolls.*

Th: *That is how you should think of yourself, as someone who is deserving of much more. You complain that Walter has disappeared, but, Allison, you must also recognize how you "disappear" from yourself. Suddenly someone like a Walter comes along and soon you no longer exist.*

A: *Does this mean it is my fault?*

Th: *In no way is his behavior your fault. No man has the right to mistreat you, offer promises that he can't keep, lie to you, and not respond to you and your concerns.*

A: *Thank you. I'll talk to you next week.*

Th: *Yes, Thursday at 4 p.m. your time.*

A: *Great. Talk to you then.*

Th: *Bye now.*

Discussion

Allison is not alone. She represents a number of women who suddenly begin to question their existence. It is quite healing and therapeutic for the woman to understand that much of her feelings of self-doubt and insecurity do not emanate from her. This is a typical case of how a borderline male will use projective identification to massively infuse his own nonexistent self into the woman, and how someone like Allison will readily identify and internalize that which is projected into her.

DIFFERENT KINDS OF BORDERLINES

Just as I noted eight different kinds of narcissists in the previous chapter, I also describe eight different kinds of borderlines (Lachkar 2010). The differences between them depend on the degree to which the grandiose invades or infects the parameters of the borderline's personality structure. Many borderlines are first cousins to their narcissistic counterparts and are continually prone to emotional crisis. As Grotstein (2002) so aptly points out, "The borderline is nothing more than a failed narcissist." Again, there is considerable overlap among the different types of borderlines described below. However, these parameters at least provide us with some useful guidelines for distinguishing qualitative differences among borderlines.

The Pathological Borderline

The pathological borderline is the least toxic of the borderlines. These borderlines are basically confused rather than intentionally cruel and sadistic like malignant borderlines. Generally not abusive or destructive to themselves or others, pathological borderlines operate at a more primitive level that is characterized by delusions, distortions, magical thinking, and projective identification. Their major defenses are projective identification (*I will do to you what others have done to me!*) and splitting, which contributes to the confusion and chaos in their world. Pathological borderlines are hard to live and deal with. Many are not deliberately cruel; rather, they are simply "unaware"! *He just doesn't get it!* Their often outwardly unresponsive behavior is frustrating, and their projections stir up the V-spots in others. These projections include the typical borderline feelings of shame, guilt, and envy. The pathological borderline does not regard needs as dirty or disgusting; instead he feels persecuted and suffocated by them.

The Malignant Borderline

The malignant borderline has many similarities to the malignant narcissist. Both are characterized by extreme paranoid and antisocial behaviors. Both share defects in intimacy compounded with destructive and uncontrollable aggression. And both share severe superego defects with basically no sense of conscience or morality. Under the guise of a cause, they can act out the most heinous crimes against humanity. They are often the abusers, the molesters, the malevolent tyrannical leaders, and serial killers. The main difference is that the malignant leader has a "cause," or at least the guise of a "cause" for his outrageous aggression, whereas the serial killer has no cause other than revenge. The need to get revenge, to retaliate becomes more pervasive than life itself (Lachkar 2011).

The main difference between the pathological borderline and the malignant borderline is that the pathological borderline does not believe his presence is of importance. (*Well, I didn't call her back because I didn't think I was important enough and did not think my call to her would make a difference.*) In contrast, the malignant borderline will prove his existence through acts of sadism and violence.

The Depressive Borderline

The depressive borderline should not be confused with a person who has clinical depression. This borderline condition is often linked to early loss of an object that has never been mourned. This type of borderline is characterized by hatred turned inward toward the self. This is not to be confused with the pathological borderline, whose self-hatred is turned outward.

The Obsessive-Compulsive Borderline

At a higher level, the obsessive–compulsive borderline has a more developed and well-integrated ego, a better tolerance for anxiety and impulse control, as well as an extremely strict but well-integrated superego. At the lower level of functioning, obsessive-compulsives are obsessed with orderliness, cleanliness, and perfectionism. They are workaholics, are devoid of feelings, and invariably cannot tolerate the emotional needs or desires of others. They keep their partners on hold and never have enough time for them. They confuse needs/emotions with dirt and disgust, and will do anything to avoid intimacy.

The Antisocial Borderline

The antisocial borderline will go to any lengths to gain power, wealth, and fame. They will lie, cheat, embezzle, and even harm those closest to them. The main difference between the antisocial borderline and the other types of borderlines is that the antisocial doesn't have a conscience; nor do they feel remorse. When caught being devious or destructive, they only feel badly about being caught, but not for the damage or sorrow they have caused others.

The Passive-Aggressive Borderline

The passive-aggressive personality type no longer exists in the DSM-IV. However, for our purposes, I have resurrected this disorder. There are many similarities between the passive-aggressive and the pathological borderline. Both disappear through a nonexistent self. The pathological borderline gains a sense of existence through projective identification, coercing others to feel and experience what they are experiencing. Passive-aggressive types do things just to evoke anger in their partners. These are what I refer to as the baby husbands, the couch potatoes, the males who will coerce their partners and others into the parent/child dyad. They are the "mañana" husbands, the "I'll do it tomorrow" husbands.

The passive-aggressives are the most difficult to treat because in their covert, insidious way, they evoke rage in their objects. *It is not I who is the angry one! It is you! Look I didn't do anything wrong. I just forgot to pick up the tickets. No big deal!* They also set them up to take over all responsibilities. They are the ones who forget, get delayed, get sick, get lost, and often can't remember the directions to the therapist's office. Compared to the narcissist, who uses people because he feels entitled, the passive-aggressive uses people to project his repressed rage (Lachkar 2011).

The Histrionic Borderline

The histrionic exhibits an excessive display of emotions, exaggerates events, cries/laughs at a whim, and needs to be the center of attention. Histrionics are not only highly emotional, but they "become" their emotions. *I feel; therefore I am!* This is similar to the depressive borderline, who both feels depressed and becomes the depression. The histrionic's clingy, glue-like tendencies and parasitic dependency needs (often psychosomatic), combined with seductive and provocative behaviors, denote very strong borderline characteristics.

The Schizoid Borderline

The schizoid borderline's primary defense is a pervasive pattern of detachment. They have few close friends, and appear indifferent to the praise or criticism of others. Unlike the schizoid narcissist, who withdraws, the borderline schizoid retreats from his objects, thus blocking himself from any emotional involvements.

The Paranoid Borderline

The most pervasive occurrence in love relations is the discontinuity between the self and the love object when paranoid anxieties overshadow the capacity for a loving relationship. Suspiciousness, lack of trust, and inability to believe they can be loved are the salient characteristics of the paranoid borderline. *You don't really love me; you are just using me!* They precipitously and impulsively jump to immediate assumptions before the ego has time to organize the data of experience. For example, a woman tells her husband, "I just know you are having an affair; you have been coming home later and later."

The Cultural Borderline

The cultural borderline will fight to the end, retaliate, or go to any extreme in order to maintain the group's collective identity. They will self-sacrifice themselves, their families, and even their children for a cause as they adhere obsessively to cultural and family traditions. These are the people who can become freedom fighters, terrorists, and suicide bombers. Our freedom is their blasphemy. An example of the cultural borderline is a Muslim man who comes to this country, marries an American woman, and expects her to follow the traditions of his country. If she goes out in public, she must wear a head cover; if she challenges him or disobeys his commands, he will punish her.

THE BORDERLINE DILEMMA FOR THERAPISTS

Both A. J. Mahari and Marsha Linehan expressed similar concerns regarding treatment of the borderline. Therapists, as well as those who work and live with this personality, find this syndrome most perplexing. The ego disturbances and poor ego functioning, compounded by primitive defenses, prevent them from maintaining healthy object relations. In a few simple words, "we are damned if we do and damned if we don't." The need to use the language of dialectics is underscored by the borderline's splitting mechanism, which attacks the ego's ability to function, observe, think, judge, and perceive.

Mrs. W. insisted that it would help if she could call a few times a day to hear my voice. We agreed until finally it got so out of hand that the phone was ringing nonstop. When I asked Mrs. W. to limit her calls, she became enraged and accused me of depriving her and going back on my word. If I try to tell her the calls are excessive, she will argue that they are not excessive, and then we get into a battle. If I tell her the calls are intrusive, she will complain that I think my contact with others is more important than my contact with her. If I overlook the above, I will feel invaded. Instead, I let her know that her need to call so often was an indication that she required more than a once-a-week psychotherapy session, and that her need for contact was healthy. Instead of getting into a battle with Mrs. W., which certainly would have been easy to do, I invited her to add an extra session. Another challenge with Mrs. W. occurs at the end of her sessions. I find myself saying endless goodbyes but to no avail. If I say goodbye and close the door, I will be besieged with calls for throwing her out. If I wait at the door for her to leave, I am besieged with endless doorknob forget-me-nots. "Oh, just one more thing! Oh, I forget to tell you." The final dilemma with Mrs. W. is the hugs. If I don't hug her, I am cold and aloof like her mother. If I do hug her, I am overstepping my therapeutic boundaries. Wherever I turn with Mrs. W., I am in a double bind.

How did I handle this borderline?

- As far as the endless telephone calls, I address the insatiable, deprived, baby part of Mrs. W., who feels that after I have given permission for her to call between sessions, I have betrayed her. In answer to being called the betrayer, I tell her that "I didn't betray you. I changed my mind. You and I are not stuck here. We have options."
- Regarding the end-of-session dilemma, I address the unconscious part of Mrs. W that sets herself up for rejection. "You know the session ends at a certain time, so you set me up to throw you out. I never want to do that. I always like to say a cordial goodbye to you."
- About the "hugs," I tell Mrs. W., "It is not that I don't want to hug you. In fact there are times I do. But you are only thinking about rejection, which doesn't allow you to see that I am trying to maintain a healthy, professional, ethical, and safe environment for both of us (ego dysfunctionality)."

Treatment options for borderlines include antidepressants and mood stabilizers. Therapists should always recommend that borderlines receive a complete psychopharmaceutical workup. In the disappearing borderline, one part desires while the other part destroys: thus, dialectical behavioral therapy is a desirable course of treatment. The therapist must address the borderline's:

- Extreme black-and-white thinking
- Self-injury, with or without suicidal behavior
- Fears of abandonment (real or imaginary)
- Chronic feelings of emptiness
- Turbulence in relationships; swift changes from idealization to hostility for no apparent reason
- High sensitivity to rejection
- Marked and persistently unstable self-image
- Rapid mood shifts

Throughout the treatment, the therapist has to pay less attention to the behaviors and actions and more acute attention to the themes. Stay with the covert communication. Listen to the words, like the thematic motif in music or poetry; stay with the feelings, the here and the now; stay with the projections (the invasion, the betrayal, the depriver). Swallow them, take them in, and transform them into a more palatable form.

Every time Joe gets hurt or feels vulnerable he has to run to the bar to meet up with his homeboys. The therapist lets him know that when his emotions and feelings get so out of hand that he has to run away to the bar that perhaps he can run to the therapeutic bar that can help him.

SUMMARY

The borderline is unique, unlike other typologies of men who disappear or suddenly vanish from relationships or intimate connections. As much as he is desirous of a bonded and intimate relationship, his primitive defenses impede the ability to get close to others. These defenses include splitting, projection, projective identification, envy, paranoid anxiety, victimization, shame/blame attacking defenses, and distortion of reality. *As much as I need and desire you, I must destroy you. The breast that I need to supply me is also envied and therefore must be destroyed.* In contrast to the narcissist, who disappears when no longer receiving the necessary narcissistic supplies, the borderline is more concerned with issues of abandonment than with success, fame, power. The borderline is preoccupied with proving a sense of existence, and through projective identification will relive and react to his own abusive, tormented childhoods within his current love relations. *Now you will know what it feels like to be tormented and abused!* The borderline dilemma offers the therapist a perfect opportunity to employ the language of dialectics to address the splitting mechanism—two roads diverged into one.

Chapter Five

The Disappearing Schizoid

The most obvious of men who disappear is the schizoid. Others can hide, cover up their agendas with charm and a false self; however, the schizoid does not have this protective mechanism. He is devoid of armor and has no emotional shield. The schizoid has an attachment disorder. He is emotionally isolated, detached, aloof, and unable to tune into the feelings and emotions of others. Because of his detachment and icy affect, he lacks the capacity to achieve social and sexual gratification. A close relationship for him invites the danger of being overwhelmed or even suffocated. People immediately sense the schizoid's distant attitude toward them, feel insecure, and are taken aback by his indifference, how he shows no interest in what other persons have to say. They may experience him as dull, boring, humorless, and uninteresting. He is unable to exhibit caring, support, or empathy for those around him.

In relationships, schizoids show no empathy or remorse for any pain they have caused. They are often described as "robots" who live within their own internal world. They are coldly indifferent; have low affect; have no desires, needs, feelings; and have very little interest in social or interpersonal relationships. Typically, they take little pleasure in activities, have few close friends, and are indifferent to either praise or criticism from others. Their object bonds go back to an early attachment to a maternal object that was either smothering or, at the other end of the spectrum, was distant, detached, and unavailable. According to Vaknin (2011), schizoid personalities have a very limited emotional repertoire and express themselves awkwardly, hesitantly, and intermittently. They appear cold, flat, and zombie like.

It is very easy to confuse narcissists with schizoids. Both have the tendency to withdraw and live within their own worlds. There are some definitive distinctions, however. The schizoids withdraw because they are loners, social recluses who are not interested in the feelings or opinions of others. Narcissists, on the other hand, will withdraw out of arrogance, hurt feelings, being misunderstood, not feeling properly mirrored, or when they run out of narcissistic supplies. They are very much concerned with the opinion of others. According to Vaknin (2007), narcissists are people in love with themselves and withdraw from others because they no longer have use for them as mirroring self-objects.

I recall seeing one of my first schizoid patients and immediately starting to feel very uncomfortable. He exhibited no emotion, engaged in no eye contact, and was silent for most of the session. He spent most of the time looking around the room, mainly at the books on the shelf. I tried to interact with him, but found he was indifferent to everything I said. There was no reaction, no emotion—not to insight, not to praise, and certainly not to advice. When I asked him where he was or what he was thinking about, he replied, "Nothing!" Although this male did not disappear physically, I felt I was talking to an automaton.

Fairbairn (1940) linked this kind of emotional detachment that characterizes the schizoid personality to a preoccupation with inner reality rather than outer reality. He describes an overevaluation of intellectual pursuits as a means for the schizoid to avoid relating to his external objects. Bowlby (1969) stressed the important distinction between withdrawal and detachment. Detachment in the schizoid is not to be confused with withdrawal in someone like a narcissist, which stems from feeling narcissistically injured. Withdrawal is a healthier state of development since at least the person maintains a certain amount of libidinal affect. When one detaches, one goes into a state of despondency—the same kind of childlike state that occurs in children who are left alone or ignored by missing or absent parents. The infant cries out for a parent, but there is no response (Lachkar 2004b, 2008b, 2009).

I was so embarrassed. We were at a reception, a staff party where he was to meet many of my friends and colleagues. There he stood, icy cold. When they reached over to shake his hand, he pulled away. As they tried to engage him in conversation, he just stood there, totally disinterested in anything that anyone had to say, let alone what was going on around him.

Vaknin (2011) refers to the schizoid as an "inverted narcissist," one who lives vicariously through others, yet remains a recluse, uninterested in social contacts. In fact, schizoids are total loners and avoid intimate personal contact. They could not care less about what people think of them, while the narcissists engage in social contacts as part of their endless search for acceptance, approval, and objects that can mirror their grandiose self. When personally injured, the schizoid detaches from his object world. Instead of relating to external objects, the schizoid develops an unconscious attachment to his internal ones—for example, the suffocating mother, the withdrawing mother, and the detached mother. In intrapersonal relations the attachment to the schizoid's inner world becomes so intense that it completely overshadows not only his reality but his relationships with others, blocking any new experiences from developing. The more attached he becomes to his internal world, the more empty and isolated he becomes.

Many schizoids at the onset of a relationship may appear charming, seductive, and, under certain circumstances, even sexual. It is only later when feelings of intimacy, vulnerability, and dependency emerge that he typically disappears in the relationship. A common experience with the schizoid is to equate intimacy with feelings of endangerment, mainly engulfment and suffocation by women. The women he relates to are often puzzled as to how someone who seems very interested in them can suddenly become hollow, cold, indifferent, and affectless, or what pop culture refers to as the misogynist male.

The schizoid is similar to the borderline in that they both suffer from attachment disorders and experience difficulty in an early bonding experience. Both maintain a fusion with a maternal object they have never separated from. The main difference is in their affective bonding experiences. The borderline has a deep need for bonding. The schizoid is a borderline without the emotionality. Even though the borderline has a faulty bonding experience, at least the desire is there, as opposed to the schizoid, who is unaware of the need for external objects and connections to others.

Although the names sound alike, and they might have some similar symptoms, schizoid personality disorder is not the same thing as schizophrenia. Many people with schizoid personality disorder can function fairly well. They tend to choose jobs that allow them to work alone, such as night security officers and library or laboratory workers. The disappearing schizoid male may make many attempts to marry and to form relationships. Because of their reclusive nature, however, many never marry. They often end up living alone as a recluse or living with their parents in adulthood. People with schizoid personality disorder often organize their lives to avoid contact with other people. Following are some outstanding traits of people with schizoid personality disorder.

- They distance themselves from almost all social events.
- They remain apart from others at work or choose solitary jobs and activities.
- They lack a sense of humor and are awkward around other people.
- Many are highly successful in their work, which usually does not require emotion (computers, science, etc.).

- They often withdraw from sex and prematurely end a budding relationship.
- They show no concern for others who ignore or reject them.
- They are indifferent to both praise and criticism.
- Their dreams are often of solid objects like plastic, frozen ice, glaciers—which reflect the state of their inner world.

People who are married to schizoid personalities often feel left out and puzzled that the schizoid will pay more attention to the needs of family members and completely neglect the needs of his spouse. One patient reports that her husband bought his mother a bracelet from Tiffany's and totally forget her birthday. When she confronted him, he hesitated and said in his usual awkward, stammering way, *Well, uh, she is my mother!*

Wife: *Where are you going?*

Husband: *I don't know.*

W: *You don't know where you are going? Then why do you have your coat on?*

H: *Oh, I thought I would go out for a while.*

W: *Where?*

H: *It is hot in this house.*

W: *So when you start to feel emotional, you say you feel hot and think it is the temperature that drives you away?*

H: *I don't know.*

W: *So, you have your coat on and you don't know where you are going. Except that you are going to cool off.*

H: *See you later.*

PARANOID-SCHIZOID POSITION

The paranoid-schizoid position is a fragmented position by which undigested thoughts and feelings are split off and projected through projective identification. It is an inner mental space that is felt to be safe, away from thoughts and feelings of pain, emptiness, loneliness, and abandonment. Klein viewed this position as the earliest phase of development, part-object functioning and the beginning of the primitive superego. If the child views the mother as neglectful, rejecting, and unavailable, that child grows up experiencing the mother as a bad-breast object. At a more profound level, if the schizoid experiences the mother as unavailable or suffocating, he will grow to experience her as the affectless mother. As much as he tries to detach from her, through his transformation he becomes her. *I feel cold; therefore I become the coldness. I feel hot; therefore I become the pressure cooker!* In this position, the schizoid differs from the borderline in that he does not experience the same kind of loss. Sometimes the dumped woman envies the schizoid for being void of feelings. *How can I feel such pain and he feels absolutely nothing?*

PART-OBJECT FUNCTIONING VS. WHOLE-OBJECT FUNCTIONING

It takes some time to understand what it means to relate to an "object." Obviously, Freud did not mean relating to a lamp. Moreover, how do individuals relate to one another in an object relational world? I find that the concepts of part- and whole-object functioning give significance to the disappearing male syndrome, as well as lend themselves to profound usage in clinical practice. Whole objects occur at the beginning of the depressive position, marked by the infant's awareness of his mother as a "whole object," someone who has needs and feelings, as opposed to the mother being only the provider for the child.

Women involved with the disappearing narcissist commonly experience the narcissist's unavailability: as soon as she expresses her needs, he's gone. This often brings about ambivalences. One part of her feels loved and valued, while the other is destroyed through neglect, envy, or sadistic, aggressive impulses. *I only love women who have big breasts!* In normal development the child begins to see the mother as a separate person with separate needs, feelings, and desires. However, the part-object functioning that occurs in the paranoid-schizoid position brings with it the danger of primitive idealization and only seeing the person in part—e.g., her breasts, his wallet, his power, her sexuality. This is where guilt, jealousy, control, domination and oedipal rivals become the replacement for love. When people are viewed and valued for "their parts," it is also common for them to feel "used" and devalued as human beings.

EXAMPLE OF PART-OBJECT FUNCTIONING

A brilliant, highly skilled scientist who was working on very technical projects at a jet propulsion lab and was regarded as one of their finest scientists, came into treatment, feeling lonely and depressed. He had a hard time relating to and maintaining relationships with women. As his history unfolded, he revealed having been raised by Mormon parents—a very stoic father and a mother who made him feel shame and humiliation at even the slightest mention of any attraction to girls, and later women. I had a suspicion that lurking beneath her religious beliefs was envy, an enactment of not wanting to share her brilliant son with others. After a while he reported that he just lost interest. Having any reaction to women exacted too big a price. I suddenly noticed that during each session he would wiggle his foot. It would just keep wiggling and wiggling. I finally called it to his attention to let him know that his foot was trying to tell me something: that when he was turned on to me either physically or emotionally, he would have his foot talk to me instead of his penis. And, of course, this led to an extensive exploration of his repressed sexual urges and fantasies.

The Case of Barbara

Barbara came into my office—a clinical emergency—breathless, choking, and sobbing hysterically.

He's disappeared! My old girlfriend fixed me up with a guy. We met at a bar, went out a few times. He seemed very attracted to me. We got into bed, took off our clothes. He tells me I am sexy and gorgeous. He plays around with me for a while. And just when he begins to penetrate, he jumps out of bed, puts his pants on, and leaps out the door. I tried to run after him, but he drove away. I kept asking myself what I did wrong. What did I say? Was I too pushy? I can't believe he doesn't miss me, think of me and all our wonderful experiences together. It was so special. Finally, I decided to do something about it. I tracked him down. Went to his favorite restaurants, stores, even the car wash, until I found him. I cornered him. "Well," he said, "we were just getting too close. I was madly in love once before with my college girlfriend, and suddenly she dumped me for another guy. I was devastated and I am still just fuming and boiling over. So I decided then and there I would never allow myself to get hurt again."

Barbara's story made it apparent that she was describing a wounded and damaged man who most likely was suffering from suffocation fantasies. Instead of feelings of love turning into something good, love got distorted and transformed into a boiling-hot pot—or shall we say his V-spot—that was about ready to explode. I let Barbara know that her emotions of vulnerability are healthy, especially compared to his feelings, which translate to fear and danger. "At least you did not run away from love. The healthy part of you knows how to bond and maintain an intimate relationship. He, on the other hand, just panicked and ran!"

The Case of Jerrold

Earlier it was mentioned how borderline and psychotic patients not only feel the pain but become the pain. There is a parallel with the schizoid. They do not feel or express their feeling of suffocation; rather, they actually become it. *I feel suffocated; therefore, I become the boiling pot and must evacuate.* The case of Jerrold illustrates this.

Therapist: *Hi, Jerrold. Please come in and have a seat.*

Jerrold: (looking aloof while walking into the room, making no eye contact with the therapist)

Th: (reaches out to shake Jerrold's hand; Jerrold pulls away)

J: (silence, still looking around the room)

Th: *So, Jerrold, what brings you here?*

J: *I don't know.*

Th: *It was my understanding that you are here because of your relationship with your girlfriend.*

J: *I guess so. I really don't care about the relationship. She's the one who wanted me to come here.*

Th: *Why is that?*

J: *She claims that I'm cold, distant, and that I pull away whenever we have intimacy.*

Th: *Well, I don't know too much about your situation. What I do know from talking with your girlfriend is that as soon as you get close to her or enter her vagina, you pull away. And as far as I know, you have not talked to her for several weeks. This is when she contacted me.*

J: (looking nervous, still aloof, and appearing uncomfortable and indifferent)

Th: *Jerrold, this may seem a bit premature, but I know you are here because you obviously do care about your girlfriend and want things to be better. There is something about a woman's vagina that is dangerous and threatening to you.*

J: *It is very scary. I don't know how to describe the fear, but I know it is scary. I get very hot. I feel like I can't breathe, and I just want to run away.*

Th: *Did you ever have any of those feelings before?*

J: (hesitantly) *Yes, my mother was always controlling, dominating my every move. All I remember is that I just wanted to run away.*

Th: *Jerrold, this is very helpful. What you're describing is suffocation anxiety, a suffocating internal mother. You are now feeling suffocated by your girlfriend's vagina, just as you felt suffocated by your mother's dominating, controlling, relentless voice.*

J: (a slight glimpse of recognition) *I suppose.*

Th: *I realize this is speculation, but I am trying to help you get more attached to your feelings, since you have a tendency to detach from them.*

J: *I guess so.*

Th: *So your girlfriend's vagina becomes your mother's mouth that is nonstop and smothering.*

J: *All I know is that as soon as I entered her vagina, I had to run.*

Th: *If I may, I would like to make one more comment, and then we will continue this next week. It does seem to me, Jerrold, that you have formed an attachment with an internal suffocating mother that interferes with your capacity to have a healthy intimate relationship with your girlfriend.*

J: *Uh-huh.*

Th: *On a precautionary note, I would recommend that next time you have these feelings, instead of fleeing try to use your words to express them. It is okay to tell your girlfriend that you feel uncomfortable, suffocated, and that she should not take your indifference personally. You may not be aware how very hurtful this is for her.*

J: *Okay, doctor. Thank you very much. I am glad this session is over.*

Th: *I understand, because I'm sure that you may be having the same feelings here, that my voice may be suffocating you. See you next week.*

Discussion

Jerrold is a perfect illustration of the disappearing male. He typifies the schizoid personality, one who is perceived as strange, cold and detached, and feels suffocated and engulfed by women. He internalizes her body parts and her emotions as dangerous, persecutory, and threatening. His history, emanating from childhood, reveals a pervasive pattern of detachment from an affectless mother. In this case, the therapist takes a very aggressive role, almost feeding words into him. Since Jerrold's emotions are basically unmentalized, the therapist feels justified in verbalizing and speculating what his feelings might be. His feelings become the heat, the vagina becomes his mother's mouth, and intimacy becomes equated with smothering. The therapist is somewhat precipitous in her speculations and risks overstepping the boundaries. However, she feels she at least must attempt to provide an opportunity for Jerrold to make sense out of the senselessness and help bring meaning to the meaningless.

THE SCHIZOID VS. THE ANTISOCIAL

Although they are two completely different entities, there can be considerable overlap between the schizoid and the anti-social. Both have a tendency to be loners and tend to socially withdraw. The antisocial can use his knowledge and social savior-faire to charm and lure people. However, he has no conscience and takes advantage of his victims by stealing, lying, or misguiding them. Bernie Madoff, who pulled off a massive Ponzi scheme that duped people out of millions of dollars, is a good example of an antisocial personality. The schizoid, on the other hand, lacks charm and social graces, has no close friendships, and is indifferent to the feelings of others. Ted Kaczynski, known as the Unabomber, was diagnosed by several forensic psychiatrists as a paranoid schizophrenic; others saw him as schizoid, a very angry man who suddenly "blows." What is noteworthy is that after their acts of destruction both Madoff and Kaczynski showed no feelings of remorse. The schizoid is split off from emotions, whereas the antisocial has no conscience at all.

We often hear horror stories of young men who have no history of violence or criminal record but will suddenly lash out and kill or bomb people at random. In fact, as I was writing this section on the schizoid, James Holmes entered a movie theater in Aurora, Colorado, and opened fire. It was a random shooting spree that ultimately claimed the lives of 12 innocent men, women, and children (CNN News, July 20, 2012).This took place at a premiere showing of *The Dark Knight Rises.* Holmes, who was dressed in black and wore a helmet, body armor, a gas mask, and a groin protector, entered the theater through a side door. His aim was not just to kill but to terrorize.

Certainly not all schizoids are terrorists and killers. But many experts confirm that loners who are unable to maintain friendships, are reclusive, and have no close bonds are at higher risk for acting out these horrific random killings. Both Ted Kaczynski and James Holmes fit the bill. They were isolated, brilliant, and highly educated men with sterling academic credentials from well-known universities. But both also were very angry men, developmentally living in the paranoid-schizoid position. Theoretically, one could reason that schizoids are people whose emotions build up, begin to simmer, get hotter and hotter until, having no outlet to express them, they finally explode.

Another possibility is the lack of identity and, in the case of Holmes, having a fixation on Batman and The Joker, thus facilitating identification with an aggressive figure and providing justification for committing such a heinous crime. *I didn't do it; the Joker did!* Someone like Holmes differs from a mass murderer. They have a history of depression, have no record of prior problems, and do not fit into society. They eventually disengage from any previous endeavors and interests, and suddenly become consumed with the need for revenge and for punishing a society that has not made a place for them. They feel their only recourse is to attack.

KLEIN'S FORMULATION ON CRIMINALITY

Klein's pioneer work on criminality in children (1927) provides the perfect impetus for children who are inclined toward schizoid personality and antisocial disorders. Often these children have been severely inhibited and not allowed the freedom to express themselves or develop a fantasy world. In her pioneering work in play therapy, Klein noted early on that there were some children who were not allowed to express their rageful, hostile, murderous impulses. She allowed children to explore these fantasies by attacking toy images of men, women, children, and animals, and to freely mutilate, kill, beat, cut, and slice them to act out their aggressive and sadistic impulses. Through play therapy, the child is able to distinguish the act of "doing" and the act of fantasizing about doing it. In other words, it is okay to fantasize about killing and mutilating mommy's breasts or daddy's penis, but it is not okay to do it. What would Melanie Klein say to James Holmes as a child while he was collecting toy guns and bomb material to booby trap his house? *Oh, I see you like to play with guns and weapons that can kill and destroy people. Okay, let's do it together and play out that fantasy.*

SUMMARY

This chapter described, defined, and outlined the defenses, behaviors, and characteristics of the schizoid, with the intent of helping therapists provide solace and comfort for the dumped woman. Women who have been abandoned feel devastated and traumatized by these men because they are inclined to identify and personalize the situation without taking into consideration that they were never dumped. The schizoid never bonded with them in the first place. He was emotionally incapable of doing that. Although we don't need to give these women a detailed explanation of the psychological make-up of schizoid personality, it is important to educate them so they can disidentify with the negative projections the schizoid unconsciously transmits to them through projective identification. *Now you will know what it feels like to have an affectless, detached mother!* At the more severe end of the spectrum, is the type of schizoid who appears to be innocent and high functioning and then suddenly blows. Teachers, counselors, professors, co-workers, family members have no clue how one can suddenly commit such horrific crimes as James Holmes did. Makes one think: If all these people didn't know what was going on in the schizoid mind, how could the women he gets involved with possibly know?

Chapter Six

The Disappearing Obsessive-Compulsive

The Robotic Male

So far we have discussed a variety of men with personality disorders, and how each type has its own unique ways of "disappearing": the narcissist through withdrawal, the borderline through splitting and projective identification, and the schizoid through withdrawing entirely from his object world. Now we turn to the obsessive-compulsive, one who does not disappear physically and, in fact, remains quite solid, almost an immovable object. The disappearance here refers to emotional/intrapsychic withdrawal.

Just as I refer to the schizoid as the hollow man, I refer to the obsessive-compulsive as the robotic man, for he operates from a different wiring system. He is pre-programmed to ward off anything that he perceives as dirt, mess, confusion, or chaos. Everything must come in a neat and tidy package. Ironically, as much as these personality types value order they become the messer-uppers. These are the collectors, the hoarders, the ones so obsessed with time and order that they often cannot even make an appointment on time. I am reminded of a lawyer, who spent so much time filing, counting, wiring the outdoor gate to ensure it was double locked, and putting things in order that by the time he checked the doors, the alarm and went through obsessive routines for leaving the house, he would arrive in court late, causing humiliation for himself and his client.

The difference between how the narcissist and the obsessive-compulsive disappear is that the narcissist fluctuates between withdrawal and need for the self-object. By comparison, the obsessive-compulsive withdraws not out of need for the self-object but for the objects themselves (work, books, files, boats, computers, technology). An example is the narcissist and the obsessive-compulsive who walk into a restaurant and order. The narcissist's repeated demands that the waiter exchange the food because it is not perfect enough differ from the obsessive-compulsive's demands to exchange the food. The narcissist feels entitled to take advantage, whereas the obsessive-compulsive fears contamination (e.g., the mashed potatoes must be apart from the fish).

The obsessive-compulsive is driven by a very harsh, punitive, and relentlessly demanding superego. Although he differs from the antisocial (who has no conscience), the obsessive-compulsive also has very little regard or concern for others, and is preoccupied with work ethics, principles, and causes. Under the guise of a cause he can put on his withdrawing act and reappear only when it suits him. Obsessive-compulsives can be the pack rats, the hoarders, the collectors (wires, papers, rocks, newspapers). Since they bond more with objects than people they clutter their space, leaving no room for others. On a more positive note, because of their obsession with work, many are very high-functioning and successful professionals (lawyers, doctors, professors). The objects they covet and hoard become the replacement for intimacy and love. *Oh, I can't get rid of this stuff. These things bring back so many memories.*

FLAWED PARTNERSHIPS

Paradoxically, obsessive-compulsive men often choose histrionic or dependent, emotional, over-the-top partners. These are women who are overly emotional, loud, messy, disorganized, and often dysfunctional. *I am a reserved kind of a guy, and whenever we go somewhere she embarrasses and humiliates me. She dresses provocatively and always has to be the center of attention.*

In *How to Talk to a Narcissist* (Lachkar 2008b), I describe the dance between the obsessive-compulsive and the histrionic, how each one needs the other to play out undeveloped parts and unconscious fantasies. He needs more of her emotionality, which he long ago abandoned, and she needs more of his structure and orderliness. But as much as he needs her, he must attack her and destroy her. *All he does is attack, criticize me, and pick on me. He expects me to be perfect like him. Often he just storms out of the house. Sometimes I don't see him for days. When he returns, he stays up night after night working. He just disappears! This is when I lose it and get totally hysterical. I start screaming, cussing, and yelling, but he just phases me out, does not listen or pay any attention to any of my feelings. He just continues on hacking away at the computer 'til all hours of the night.*

The obsessive-compulsive man has a delusional inner emotional experience. To him emotions, feelings, and desires are something dirty, crawly, destined to contaminate or infect a perfect world. These are the men who are obsessed with cleanliness and have a delusional sense of the dangers of "dirt." They will compulsively wash their hands again and again, check and recheck doors, file and re-file, and organize cabinets to ensure orderliness and sanitation. These are the men who confuse love, emotions, and vulnerability with something so filthy that it is only suitable for evacuation. It must be gotten rid of. The obsessive-compulsive man (or woman) cannot tolerate confusion, chaos, confrontation, or anything that stirs up a perfectly cleansed internal world. When their perfect world is tampered with, they defend in two ways. First, they withdraw into a robotic state, and, second, they clean, file, and do everything possible to restore order, often creating internal chaos and turmoil in the process. Of course, it is not fair to classify all obsessive-compulsives this way, but where relational love bonds are concerned, there does seem to be a certain cluster of men who share these common defenses.

It is usually at this juncture where women get very discouraged at trying to pull out some emotionality from the obsessive-compulsive: *Did you miss me? Do you love me? How do you feel about me?* Because needs are felt to be dirty and these men aim to live in a sterile, dirt-free environment, when pressured to express their feelings, they flee (usually only momentarily because of the pressure they feel to return to their work). *I have had enough of your emotions, needs, and demands!* They are every environmentalist's dream since they are usually the first to contribute to environmental causes and always put trash in the correct collectible containers. They're solidly "green."

Wife: *You already washed your hands!*

Husband: *I want to be sure I don't catch a cold.*

W: *But you have already washed your hands three times!*

H: (no reply)

W: *You know, Mr. Perfect, we are going to be late to the theater. And for someone who has to be perfect, don't you think we should try to be on time?*

H: *I am always on time.*

W: *Not last week when we were invited to dinner. By the time you checked the doors, locked up your files, found a tie without a stain, and washed your hands we were late.*

H: *That's because you were badgering me. That is why we were late. What do you want me to do? Leave the house without checking the doors, the lights, the oven?*

W: *So checking everything ten times is more important than respecting our friends? You always place more importance on objects than people.*

H: *If I left it up to you, the house would have been burned down.*

W: *You could use a little fire, especially in our love making. You are cold and aloof and never express any emotions.*

H: (withdrawing) *Yep, that's me!*

Obsessive-compulsives often have mothers of two varieties. The first is the mother who does not allow her child to express emotions and inhibits and represses any feelings the child may have. They are often the mothers who toilet trained their children much too soon and taught them early on that their feces are bad and dangerous. This is where feelings are translated into dirt and shame. These are the anal mothers, the withholding mothers, mothers more concerned with perfection than love and closeness. The second type is the overly emotional mother, the one who yells, screams, is messy, suffocating, and clingy. She drives her son to develop a manic defense in order to become the opposite of her. *I will show her how disgusting she is by having nothing to do with her. I am now a robot!* The irony is that in spite of the obsessive-compulsive's intent to become the opposite of his mother and thinking he has mastered the art of separation-individuation, he has not only not separated from her, he is fused. He becomes a caricature of her and then finds as an object choice someone exactly like her.

COMMON COMPLAINTS ABOUT THE OBSESSIVE-COMPULSIVE

- He is too domineering and controlling.
- He neglects and me and never has time for me.
- He puts everything first—his work, his sports, his friends, etc.
- He makes me feel worthless, as though everything is more important than our kids and our family.
- He makes me feel like my needs, desires, and feelings are insignificant and hateful.
- He makes me feel like my emotions will endanger him or contaminate him.
- He makes me crazy when he takes forever to leave the house or finish getting dressed.

- He always has to be right, and I am always wrong.
- He always turns things I say about him against me.

Typically, the obsessive-compulsive remains forever attached to his mother's body. He believes he has separated from her, but fusion with the maternal object is manifested by finding a woman like the mother or the exact opposite of her. The obsessive-compulsive has a self that has been long ago abandoned, a lost self that is devoid of feelings and emotions and operates to repel the mother or to find a partner that exhibits the same attributes of the mother. *Who wants to be emotional like my mother. I find her needs to be repulsive. So when I listen to my wife express feelings, I must admit that I don't hear her; I hear the voice of my wailing mother!*

The Case of Fred and Margaret

This couple has been married for fifteen years and has three children. She is a surgical nurse, and he a successful entrepreneur. Fred comes in with well-groomed hair, wearing a spotlessly clean Ralph Lauren shirt, perfectly pressed Dockers, matching belt, and Rolex watch. Margaret is wearing shorts that are not ironed, a wrinkly green T-shirt, and worn-out tennis shoes. Her hair is unkempt. Margaret's presenting complaint is that Fred is always on her case—in the kitchen, in the car, in the bedroom—and that he does not stop picking on her and attacking her. She complains that he is Mr. Perfect and wants her to be exactly like him. When she rebels, he takes off for his boat, his work, his charities, his causes.

Therapist: *Greetings! Please have a seat.*

Fred and Margaret: *Thank you.*

Th: *Who would like to start?*

F: (looks at Margaret) *Why don't you start?*

M: *Why don't* you *start?*

F: *You're the one with all the complaints, so why don't you start?*

M: *If I start, you'll get mad at me for complaining and you'll get up and leave!*

Th: *I would not think of you as complaining. I see you instead as someone here to try to make things better.*

M: *Better! Nothing can make things better. Fred is very controlling, domineering. He cannot stand for things to be out of place. Everything has to be done his way. If I open the blinds, he immediately closes them. I can't even cook without him criticizing me or complaining.*

F: *Well, why can't you cook without getting crumbs all over the floor?*

M: *See what I mean? I can't win an argument. He thinks he's perfect and can't take any criticism. And he has plenty of dirt that he keeps swept under the carpet.*

Th: (wondering why a man who has to be so perfect would choose such a messy, unkempt, unattractive wife)

M: *All he wants to do is hike, work, go on his boat. He never thinks of me, and afterwards he is so exhausted he doesn't have time for sex.*

Th: *Margaret, you are talking about emotions, feelings, and getting your needs met, and you, Fred, seem to be all about objects, things, and perfection.*

F: *What's wrong with that?*

Th: *Nothing. But two people who are married and have children need to begin to communicate and understand each other's language* (therapist's attempt to mirror their experience).

M: *Right. He says I'm too emotional, and he wants me to stop bugging him.*

Th: *Fred, you are so perfect in so many ways. You are a great dad, a creative and resourceful entrepreneur and have developed many patents. You are also a great athlete. But when it comes to being a husband, you are not so perfect* (therapist resorts to language of empathology before she confronts him).

M: *Right on!!!*

F: *Well, at least you appreciate me and all the effort I make to support this family.*

Th: *And you, Margaret, are a very hard-working woman. You are a surgical nurse. You get up every morning at 5 a.m., have three kids, and your husband expects you not to drop any crumbs on the floor.*

F: *Yes, she is all those things. But being a nurse one would think she'd be a little neater. And she gets far too hysterical over every little thing I say.*

Th: *Fred, I think she is telling you she is being treated in a crummy way.*

F: *This is an insult. I feel like getting the hell out of here.*

Th: *Now you are doing with me what you do with your wife. Instead of taking responsibility for your part in the relationship you want to run away* (therapist inviting herself into the couple transference).

M: *Right on!! See, he thinks I am like his mother who completely dominated and controlled him.*

Th: *This is great! In just a few moments I have your "dance" choreographed right here before me. Fred, you would like your wife to be neater and less emotional, more like you. But there is a part of you that needs some of Margaret's emotionality. As for you, Margaret, you need some of Fred's structure, his orderliness, his neatness.*

F: *You're right. She gets so hysterical, I can't take it!*

Th: *Margaret, getting hysterical and out of control does make a mess. Setting boundaries and limits with Fred is not the same as setting them with your kids. If Fred criticizes, you can calmly tell him to stop. If he doesn't, then leave the room, take a break, and return when things are calm. You need more boundaries, and he needs more emotionality* (therapist helping Margaret not take in his negative projections).

F: *That would be better. At least she will get off my back.*

Th: *Yes, she can get off your back by becoming more like you, less hysterical, and you can get off her back as well by not invading her space.*

F: *I don't think I can do that.*

M: *Why not?*

Th: *Oh yes, you can!*

F: *How do you know?*

Th: *Because you are perfect!* (happy to see both partners chuckling a bit) *See you next week.*

Discussion

In this case we can see how both partners operate within the paranoid-schizoid position. Fred does not view Margaret as a whole object, a woman with needs and feeling, but rather as a part object, someone he can control and dominate. In the dance of the couple, we see how these oppositional partners stir areas of unconscious development in each other. Fred needs more of Margaret's emotionality and Margaret's needs some of Fred's structure and orderliness. As treatment unfolds it becomes clearer that Fred identifies with his controlling, domineering mother; as much as he despises her, he becomes her and then has to repudiate her. This is when he disappears!

SUMMARY

As in most of the cases presented in this book, the therapist is rather precipitous in confronting the resistances and defenses of the disappearing male. This lack of hesitation is deliberately designed to show how men with each type of disorder manifest their own unique way of disappearing or withdrawing. In reality, not too many therapists would expose the dynamics and defenses so early without first developing a bonding relationship. However, for our purposes confronting the defenses somewhat prematurely helps sharpen our awareness and makes the various ways men withdraw or disappear become more glaringly apparent. Many therapists become frustrated trying to break through the bedrock stratum of defenses. One method is through confrontation, which can be a more effective approach than an empathic stance. The main task in dealing with the obsessive compulsive, as with the other types of disappearing male, is to help women disidentify with the negative projections that the disappearing men translocate into them by giving them the necessary tools and communication skills to deal with verbal assaults and mistreatment.

Chapter Seven

The Disappearing Passive-Aggressive

Much to my dismay, passive-aggressive personality disorder was removed from the DSM-IV and relegated to an appendix mention. In this book—as well as in many of my previous publications (Lachkar 2008a, 2008b, 2010)—I have taken the liberty of resurrecting it because it fits perfectly with the behaviors and character traits of the disappearing male.

This category has significance in discussing the disappearing male syndrome, mainly because the passive-aggressive is always trying to coerce others to form a parent/child dyadic relationship. The passive-aggressive disappearing male has an undue sense of dependency and is so child-like that he uses his partner to re-create the parent/child dyad. Typically, passive-aggressives manipulate others and get them to perform functions for them by enacting the role of the victim through illness, accidents, forgetfulness, and the like. *My mommy wife will take care of everything.* Because many of these personality types have been deprived and abused in their childhoods, they feel the world owes them something, that it should take pity on them and care for them. Actually, they have a reverse sense of entitlement: they are not concerned about success, rewards, or accolades, and are more invested in forming parasitic bonds with their objects.

The way the passive-aggressive withdraws differs from withdrawal by the schizoid, the obsessive-compulsive, and many other disorders characterized in this book. The passive-aggressive is more closely aligned with the borderline personality, mainly because of the loss of reality, as well as the tendency to procrastinate and form parasitic bonds with his objects. Both are similar in that they coerce their objects under the guise of the "poor me" victim. The main distinction is that the borderline expresses his rage outwardly, while the passive-aggressive expresses his rage inwardly. The passive-aggressive is similar to the narcissist in that they both share entitlement fantasies and turn to others to perform functions for them. However, the narcissist functions at a higher level. The narcissist will use people to enhance his grandiose self, whereas the passive-aggressive could care less about grandiosity; he is more concerned about maintaining his victimized state. Both live in a delusional world, with expectations that others should assume responsibility for their well-being and live up to their unrealistic requirements.

Passive-aggressives typically procrastinate, feign incompetence, and find a plethora of excuses why they were not able to follow through. These are the couch potatoes, the promisers, the "do-it-laters," the mañana men (Lachkar 2008b). They complain that other people make unrealistic demands on them, especially with respect to authority. They defend against the demands that others make of them by pretending incompetence and forgetfulness, devaluing the significance of the task, and disavowing the needs of others. They unconsciously set up their partners and coworkers to get angry with them, while they maintain a state of innocence and purity. *Me, I didn't do anything. I just forgot my car keys.*

Furthermore, the passive-aggressive is full of repressed rage and unconscious hostility, emanating from early depriving and neglectful caretakers who were inattentive to his needs. Many of these caretakers discouraged the child's expression of anger, resulting in suppressed hostility that is dangerous and persecutory. The most frustrating thing for a woman involved with a passive-aggressive disappearing male is the way he makes endless promises, offers a stream of excuses, and never follows through. They insidiously provoke their partners to turn them into the outwardly mad and crazy ones. *Look it is you who are the angry one; all I did was fall asleep on the couch.*

Passive-aggressives are among the most difficult patients to treat because they feel trapped and paralyzed by their dependency needs and covertly drive their partners insane. They often seduce their partners, and even the well-seasoned therapist, to sympathize with them, feel sorry for them, and go along with the "bad-mommy" who has created all these demands and been cruel. In court custody cases, passive-aggressives are often the brilliant manipulators who convince judges, lawyers, and court mediators that they are innocent and mild and meek bystanders—that it is the bad wife who is causing all the conflict.

Both the therapist and partner are often left waiting, worrying, and thinking maybe something tragic has happened and are relieved when the passive-aggressive finally arrives. It is very typical for the passive-aggressive to keep everyone always wondering about them and preoccupied with them. Another way they accomplish this is to form a parasitic dependency bond. *Sorry I was late; I got stuck in traffic. I fell asleep on the couch. I'll tell you tomorrow; I haven't decided yet. Let me check out my schedule. I was not feeling well.* Yet tomorrow never comes, and the excuses never stop. The passive aggressive is frequently the product of sibling rivalry conflicts, whereby he grows up feeling deprived of maternal attachment and spends the rest of his life searching for ways to reattach. A caretaker-type woman often makes a perfect target for these types of men. *I felt so sorry for him. He lost his house. His wife took all his money and accused him of child abuse, so I could not help but want to take care of him.*

A shared common dynamic is how passive-aggressives translocate or project their repressed rage and anger into their significant others. As an aside, this is often a very common trait in the workplace, whereby employees will covertly act out their most aggressive impulses toward their employers. How does this relate to the disappearing male syndrome? The narcissistic disappears into his own world of specialness, disregarding the needs of others, while the passive-aggressive withdraws—not to ensure a sense of specialness but as a means to maintain his dependent state of mind or, more simply, to retreat into the world of "baby husbands."

The Case of Mr. and Mrs. Pastor

Therapist: *Hi! So! What brings you here?*

Mrs. Pastor: *I am so angry and frustrated.*

Th: *Oh* !

Mrs. P.: *He's impossible to live with. I can't take it anymore. He is always late, forgetful, and comes with a bunch of excuses. Meanwhile, our bills aren't paid, and he still doesn't have a job.*

Th: *How does he make excuses?*

Mrs. P.: *Last week he was supposed to meet me at a property that we were going to show clients, and he forgot the key!*

Mr. Pastor: *I did not forget the key. You told me you were going to bring it.*

Mrs. P.: I *did not. It was your responsibility and your fault that the clients couldn't get into the house.*

Mr. P.: *You are always blaming things on me.*

Mrs. P.: *Of course, I blame you. Why shouldn't I? You always pick up the kids late from school and forget to pick up food at the grocery store. So when I come home there is nothing in the house to eat. When I ask you where you want to go, what you want to eat, or what movie you want to see, I always get the same response: "Whatever" or "I don't know."*

Mr. P.: *Do you see how she blames me and picks on me for everything? The reason I was late to pick up the kids was because I thought they had soccer practice.*

Th: *This is not about finding fault and blame. As we can see, this becomes like a dance that goes round and round without stopping. It never reaches any conflict resolution.*

Mrs. P.: *Then what do you suggest?*

Th: *I suggest we look at the couple dynamics. Mrs. P., you are not talking about a grown man, but a little-boy husband who sets you up to play the bad-breast mommy role. And you, Mr. P., are setting your wife up to express the anger that you never learned how to express. It reminds me of what you said about your mother—how she never allowed you to express anger or disappointment.*

Mr. P.: *What the hell are you talking about? Calling me a kid and a baby husband? What the fuck gives you the right?* (Mr. P goes on a rampage)

Mrs. P. and Th: (remain silent)

Th: *I think this is wonderful!*

Mrs. P.: *Wonderful! What do you mean "wonderful"? The guy has lost his mind!*

Th: *This is the only time in treatment when I actually encourage this kind of aggression. How great that the anger comes out directly rather than in an insidious or subversive fashion like forgetting, feigning weakness, making excuses, etc.*

Mrs. P.: *I never would have thought about it in this way before—encouraging his rage.*

Th: *Nobody has ever thought about encouraging his anger. It's been suppressed his whole life.*

Mr. P.: *No one in my family ever allowed me to get angry, to express my feelings. I always had to be the good little boy.*

Th: *I really don't like you swearing at me or your wife, but at this point it is preferable to expressing your rage silently and stirring up rage in your partner or me. I know it is not easy for you, but while you are here you have an opportunity to express yourself directly because, unlike your mother, this is the healthy part of you.*

Mrs. P.: *Is it always going to be like this here: him ranting all the time?*

Th: *Of course not. We are just beginning to open up a new space in which you can express your feeling in a civilized manner. But it will take time. You both did very well. See you next week.*

Mr. P.: *Can I pay you next week? I forgot my checkbook.*

Th: (smiling) *Yes, of course. See you both then.*

Discussion

This case is a good example of how patients move through various stages of treatment (see chapter 11). Mr. and Mrs. P. are clearly in the first phase of treatment (the paranoid-schizoid position). In this phase it is important for the therapist to have empathic attunement with both partners (listening, showing authority, determining the timing). Yet Mr. P., who was more inclined toward borderline pathology, allowed the therapist to be more confrontational. The therapist intuitively knew what would incur his wrath. At the end of the session when Mr. P. said he forgot the check, the therapist made the judgment call to let it pass and not make this an issue, even though she could easily have said, "Now you are forgetful with me!" Although it would have marked the beginning of opening up to the couple transference, it would not have been good timing and could have interfered with the main focus of the session—the insidious way that Mr. P. projected his rage. The therapist purposely held back getting into the couple transference until the couple moved further along. The therapist also chose not to push the boundaries too early—for example: "If your husband forgets to pay the bill, then the bill doesn't get paid. If your husband is late to the theater, then go without him." To push the boundaries in the very early stage of treatment would have been precipitous, but eventually the therapeutic challenge is to relieve the woman of her caretaking role. It is also noteworthy that the therapist purposely referred to the husband as Mr. P. rather than by his first name. This was done to remind him of his adult/male status.

THE BABY HUSBAND

Many women claim they see passive-aggressive men as baby husbands. In psychological terms they are referring to men who have not overcome or mastered their oedipal complex or their oedipal rivals. To feel safe in father's house, one must first have a secure relationship and attachment with the mother.

Mrs. A. comes into session crying and feeling very upset. "My husband never tells me when he is coming home. He says one time and then shows up three hours later. He manufactures all kinds of excuses. Then when I ask him what he would like for dinner, he responds with the famous words, 'I don't know.' When I corner him into answering me, he says his other favorite line, 'Whatever!' I said, 'If I ever hear the word whatever from you again I am going to scream.'"

The above example is typical of the kinds of predicaments the disappearing passive-aggressive puts his partner through. In relationships the passive-aggressive will generally choose an obsessive-compulsive type with a sharp sense of responsibility, who feels it is her obligation to take care of others. Obsessive-compulsive personalities are also dependent and subjugate their own needs to those of others. They are the ones who readily introject the passive-aggressive's victimization and feel responsible for them. I am reminded of a woman who had eight younger siblings and was made responsible for them at a young age; her mother made her a "little adult" much too soon. *Sometimes I feel as though my husband is my younger brother, helpless and powerless, and I must care for him.*

Below is an example of how a passive-aggressive man can coerce a woman into taking over the caretaker role at the very onset.

A passive-aggressive man calls a woman for a first date and says he would like to meet her. She responds by saying, "Sure that would be wonderful." He keeps repeating how much he would like to meet her, but never sets a definite date. Finally out of frustration she asks, "When would you like to meet?" To this he responds, "Let me call you later." The next day he calls again, and she finally says, "Where would you like to meet?" He responds, "Anywhere." She suggests, "Why don't you let me know where, and I will meet you." He responds, "I don't know any places in West LA." She is surprised. "But I thought you lived in LA for 30 years." He replies, "But I don't go out very much."

Some of the signs of passive-aggressive behavior include:

- Makes promises that are never fulfilled
- Resents authority
- Sabotages those who care about him or try and help him
- Cannot ask directly for help (parasitic dependency)
- Projects victimization and coerces others to pity him and do things for him
- Has unresolved oedipal issues and fears of intimacy at a level of maturity (the "Baby Husband")
- Maintains the role of the inferior male
- Exhibits chronic lateness, forgetfulness
- Creates chaos and confusion
- Complains persistently of personal hardship, illness, misfortune
- Is unable to take personal responsibility
- Has tendency to blame others for his own shortcomings
- Cannot express anger directly; instead projects it into others

TREATMENT

The passive-aggressive is one of the most difficult types of patients to treat for they are always trying to re-create the child/parent dyad. No matter how sensible or reasonable the advice given to them is, they repudiate it in order to maintain their infantile status. They are preprogrammed to disregard authority, resent people telling them what to do and what is "good for them," and refuse to heed the advice of others. They are the silent nonconformists, which explains why many have difficulty maintaining relationships, jobs, and interpersonal relations. Unlike the borderline, where unleashed anger becomes a major therapeutic threat and the therapist must nip the aggression before it explodes, with the passive-aggressive anger is actually encouraged (within limits, of course). *Anger in our family was simply not allowed. Whenever I got angry, my father would beat me with his belt and my mother would say, "Now you have something to cry about!"* The treatment approach requires the therapist to confront the aggression while showing empathy toward the anxiety but not toward the behavior.

SUMMARY

Many capable, intelligent, high-functioning women come into treatment telling their stories of heartbreak. The faces are different but the scenarios are the same. They feel they have been tricked, manipulated, suckered into falling for men who took advantage of their nurturing and caretaking character. It is important for the therapist to reassure the woman that her role as caretaker is a meaningful one and in no way should be dismissed. But it can backfire, making her a perfect target for the passive-aggressive's projections as he looks to her as the perfect, all-encompassing, feeding mommy. The woman believes that "because I am so warm, loving, and nurturing, he will appreciate me and heal from all the wounds from his past." Ironically, the opposite occurs. The passive-aggressive misinterprets the woman's nurturing and caretaking qualities as weakness, part of himself that he identifies with. As treatment progresses the therapist should look for the opportunity to introduce the woman to her internal object—the grandiose, neglected part of herself that overlooks her own needs and is overly compliant to the needs of others.

As with so many couples I describe in *The Narcissistic/Borderline Couple* and other publications (2004, 2008a, 2008b, 2011), in treating the dance between the passive-aggressive and his caretaker, the therapist must be acutely aware of the overlapping dynamics between containment on the part of the caretaker and self-expression on the part of the passive-aggressive. *Just as your husband has difficulty expressing his anger, you have difficulty suppressing and containing your grandiose self, which interferes with getting your own needs met. It puts you in the compromising position of an enabler, a receptacle for his evacuations and projected rage.* The therapist is now in the strategic position to do deeper analytic work, pointing out how each partner not only identifies with the negative projections of the other but over-identifies with them, which I ascribe to dual projective identification.

Chapter Eight

The Disappearing Depressive

The exact cause of depression is not known. Many researchers believe it is caused by chemical changes in the brain due to genetics or triggered by certain stressful events. More likely, it's a combination of both. Difficulties in diagnosing depression include discerning how much is genetic and how much is environmental or from social pressures and strains. While some types of depression can be traced through family genetics, others do not play a part in family history.

There are many different kinds of depression: normal depression, major depressive disorder/clinical depression, unipolar depression, borderline depression, bipolar depression, and psychotic depression. Among these is Melanie Klein's (1957) formulation of the depressive position that is considered to be healthy, connoting normal states of sadness and expression of remorse. The aim of this chapter is to illustrate how these forms of depression contribute to the disappearing male syndrome.

The most obvious form of disappearance is associated with those who have a chemical or major depression, who are suicidal, and literally disappear. Then there is the more subtle form of disappearance—the man who withdraws into an inner world of unremitting sadness is attacked by the blues and makes other people feel sad and miserable with him. Also within this cluster we have the depressive-masochist and the depressive sadomasochist. The depressive masochist is the master of self-inflicted punishment, someone who functions like a reverse narcissist and who inflicts pain against the self. The sadistic depressive, on the other hand, inflicts pain and cruelty onto others to rid the self of internal, intolerably painful affects. *Now it is you that is hurting, not me. You will know what it feels like to have been abandoned and abused!*

I refer to the depressive male as a reverse narcissist, someone who withdraws outwardly and turns inward against the self. The narcissist is constantly on the search for self-mirroring objects, whereas the depressive shows a complete lack of interest in others and in normal social activities. He is completely preoccupied to the exclusion of the needs and concerns of others (Lachkar 2008a, 2008b). Most people do not realize it is aggression that runs in the opposite direction which impels the depressive to coerce others to pity, feel sorry for, and collude with their states of helplessness. A grandiose self gives the depressive a sense of entitlement to deprive the self, as well those around him. The depressive differs from the depressed narcissist in that narcissistic pathology is linked to the depletion of narcissist supplies. In contrast, the depressive does not care about narcissistic supplies or those who offer gratification or admiration; he is more invested in masochistic bonding via pain, victimization, self-flagellation, and self-blame.

The depressive male is similar to the depressive borderline male. The difference is that the depressive borderline male bonds with his objects through pain and parasitic dependency, whereas the depressive male withdraws and does not reach out for human contact. Depressed people are often uninterested in normally pleasant social activities, and may be unable to function because of lethargy or fearfulness. One man was so depressed after he was laid off from his job that he refused to see anyone, would not answer calls, and became a total recluse. His girlfriend was convinced he had broken up with her until she went over to his house and found him unshaved, drinking, and staring at the television in a stupor.

IN RELATIONSHIPS

Depressive men often hook up with borderline women who are dependent or caretaker types. Often these women do not have a sense of self and thus grasp at the feeling of being needed and wanted by their depressive partners. Because of low self-esteem, they fuse with the depressive and take in his negative projections. He reinforces her already nonexistent/abandoned self by not allowing her to provide him with any help. *Whenever I ask if he needs anything or if I can help with anything, he simply replies, "No, I don't need anything. Just leave me alone and do not bother me. No one can help me, not even you!"*

Disappearing depressive males have a great deal of difficulty with intimate relations. They are often lethargic, irritable, and critical not only of others but of themselves. They withdraw and isolate their feelings, cannot communicate or express emotions, and often back away from sexual intimacy. Many feel too shameful or undeserving to allow themselves to receive comfort and love from their partners; rather, they turn inward for consolation.

Some depressives may detach themselves from dependency needs and express them passive-aggressively or parasitically.

A major component of depression is rumination, which involves dwelling on and brooding about themes like loss and failure, which cause the person to feel even worse. The following case illustrates a man suffering from a neurotic depression and shows how the therapist helps him sort out the delusions and distortions about himself, and extend his feelings beyond his depressed state of mind. Les came into treatment referred by his physician. He immediately began to describe how helpless and powerless he felt and that there was nothing he could do about it.

The Case of Les

Therapist: *Hi, Les. Please have a seat over here, and we will begin.*

Les: *I am feeling so low, so blue and down in the dumps. I can't seem to shake myself out of it. I know I am depressed.*

Th: *So you have already diagnosed yourself?*

L: *Well, what else would you call it, doctor? I can't get up in the morning, have no appetite, and all I want to do is sleep.*

Th: *And what else?*

L: *I am experiencing depression, unless you have another name for it.*

Th: *Well, it's not clear. Depression overlaps with many other disorders. However, I am impressed that in spite of all the symptoms you mentioned, you were actually able to bring yourself to come here.*

L: *Like today. I tried to get things done and I just couldn't. So I called my girlfriend, but she never returned my call. This kind of stuff depresses me even more.*

Th: *So you felt frustrated?*

L: *Frustrated!! Everything in my life frustrates me. I haven't accomplished very much.*

Th: *That's not depression.*

L: *Well, if that is not depression, then what is it?*

Th: *Les, you are describing normal feelings of disappointment and frustration, and you have been getting a lot of mileage taking it down into the depths of depression. But basically you are dealing with loss, sadness, and frustration.*

L: *Then why do I always feel so blue, so down in the dumps?*

Th: *Because on top of feeling frustrated, abandoned, and neglected, you are punishing yourself. Self-persecution leads to a loss of reality, which you need to help you face ways of getting your life back together.*

L: *I haven't lost my reality. I know I am depressed. I feel like a nothing.*

Th: *Even now you are losing your sense of reality. Just because you feel like a nothing doesn't mean you are a nothing.*

L: *But I feel paralyzed.*

Th: *Again, that doesn't mean you are paralyzed. You seem to confuse how you feel with how things are. You even came in here today with a distorted sense of reality, thinking that you could diagnose and classify your symptoms as if you are your own therapist. The reality is that I am your therapist and I am here to help you.*

L: *You don't understand the pain I'm in.*

Th: (therapist moves now to a more empathetic stance) *I think you are right. I have not showed much empathy toward your pain and aching heart. I hear it and feel it, and it must be very difficult to live with this day after day. At the same time, I see a different person than you see, and I want to be very careful not to collude with your devaluation of yourself and your victimization.*

L: *Are you saying I am making this up?*

Th: *No, I am saying that while these feelings of disappointment, abandonment, and persecutory anxiety are operative it is hard for you to see reality, and as your therapist I have to be very careful not to collude with the distorted image you have of yourself.*

L: *Then what should I do when I can't get up in the morning to even brush my teeth?*

Th: *Crawl on your hands and knees. Know you are not paralyzed even though you feel paralyzed.*

L: *You really are trying to get me functioning, aren't you?*

Th: *Why shouldn't I? You are an intelligent, capable man and there are many opportunities for you out there.*

L: *I wish I could sound as hopeful as you.*

Th: *It is not a matter of hope. It is a matter of trying to find other work and not hiding under your depression as a way of avoidance, as you are doing with your girlfriend.*

L: I *guess I should call my girlfriend back. She will think I dumped her.*

Th: *You got it! Hang in there. See you next week.*

L: *Okay. See you then!*

Discussion

In this case the therapist takes a very confrontational stance. She initially does not show much empathy, being careful not to collude with the patient's distortions and victimized self. As a precautionary measure, the therapist is careful to remain apart from Les's distorted image of himself as downtrodden and helpless. At first Les tries to attack the therapist, attempting to make her into the helpless, useless person he feels himself to be. The therapist directs the session, addressing the grandiose and distorted image Les has of himself and showing him how he uses his depressed self to hide from intimacy. This case gives me an appreciation of how the ego becomes dysfunctional when persecutory anxiety lurks in the shadow of the psyche. As bad and painful as his state of mind is for Les, it is still better that having to face the feelings that an intimate relationship requires.

NORMAL DEPRESSION, GRIEF, AND CLINICAL DEPRESSION

Depression may be described as feeling sad, blue, unhappy, miserable, or down in the dumps, but it should not be confused with normal grief. Normal depression is in response to something tragic that occurs in everyone's life—loss of a spouse or lover, loss of a job, or the break-up of a relationship. The person will in time recover and finds enough support and ego strength to go on with his/her life. However, if extended, normal depression may lead to a major depression. Some of the symptoms of depression include:

- Agitation, restlessness, and irritability
- Withdrawal or isolation

- Difficulty concentrating
- Dramatic change in appetite, often with weight gain or loss
- Fatigue and lack of energy
- Feelings of hopelessness and helplessness
- Feelings of worthlessness, self-hate, and guilt
- Loss of interest or pleasure in activities that were once enjoyed
- Thoughts of death or suicide
- Trouble sleeping or too much sleeping

Depression that is mild and chronic is known as dysthymia, and may vary based on age or cultural factors. It is the kind of depression often linked to something as simple as a disappointment or inconvenience that may frustrate or interfere with the person's everyday life. This type of depression does not cause much emotional damage, and it usually is not lasting. Some depressive episodes last longer than others due to the severity of the cause—for example, a break-up of a relationship, a death. Yet the person is able to adapt and find resources to cope with the depression, including support groups, bereavement groups, etc.

When the depression lasts longer than approximately six months and the symptoms of sadness, withdrawal, isolation, and lack of animation are persistent, it is then considered to be a clinical depression. The person who overcomes a normal depression is considered to have a more intact ego, better coping skills, and better ability to adapt to and manage the cause of his or her depression. Women who are "dumped" by the depressed male may realize that it is only a momentary state, as opposed to those who are left by the male who is clinically depressed, in which case the relationship may not be so easily resurrected.

Although depression is often thought of as an extreme state of sadness, there is a vast difference between clinical depression and sadness. Sadness is a part of being human, a natural reaction to painful circumstances. All of us will experience sadness at some point in our lives. It is anger turned inward and against the self. While sadness is a momentary state of mind that passes as a person comes to term with his troubles, depression can linger for weeks, months, or even years.

Those suffering from depression may have a propensity toward self-harm and self-mutilation and a proclivity toward chronic suicidal ideation and acts. The depressive that operates with more severe primitive defenses not only feels the pain and wants to escape from it, but they also become the pain. *I am the pain and the pain is me!* Research findings indicate that there is not always a logical reason for one's dark feelings. Clinical depression is disabling and adversely impacts family, work, friends, and all those around the depressed person. Advice from well-meaning friends and family to "snap out of it" results only in frustration, for a clinically depressed person can no more "snap out of it" than a patient with Alzheimer's can will his brain to re-create memory. A person with clinical depression feels overwhelmed and hopeless, not merely sad. The main difference is that with normal depression reality remains intact, whereas with borderline or psychotic depression self-persecution persists and reality testing is lost.

Major depression is almost universally treated with antidepressant medication. This alternately includes psychodynamic therapy to address the underlying root of the depression, the delusions and distortion. This is often a combination of behavioral and talk therapy, supportive therapy, and DBT. For some people, a brief hospital stay can help get them on the road to recovery. Any time there is a real danger of suicide, it is wise to consider hospitalization, especially if the person does not have family and/or friends who can keep him/her safe at home.

The Case of Rick

Rick, a middle-aged stockbroker, was referred to treatment for clinical depression by a relative who noticed that he was sleeping most of the day, missing work, and skipping meals. Rick indicated that he feels paralyzed, can't move, can't function, and can hardly get up in the morning to get dressed, let alone come to therapy.

Rick: *Just got a call from my girlfriend. She broke up with me.*

Therapist: *How does this make you feel?*

R: *What do you expect? I just can't function. I just want to die.*

Th: *What happened?*

R: *She was complaining she is sick of me taking all those meds, canceling our dates, my lack of enthusiasm and zero sexual interest, my lethargy, showing no feelings for her, blah, blah, blah. I was too tired and exhausted to do anything. I thought she would have more sympathy for me and would try and be helpful.*

Th: *She did try and each time you pushed her away as if you didn't want help from her or anybody.*

R: *I just want to be left alone. Don't want anyone's help or sympathy.*

Th: *Sounds very self-destructive.*

R: *Self-destructive is right, I don't want to fight this sickness any longer. I'm done.*

Th: *Yet you seem to still have an attachment to your girlfriend. Otherwise you wouldn't have had such a strong reaction.*

R: *That's the point. I don't want to feel.*

Th: *So you hide under your depression, using it like a shield to protect yourself from feeling.*

R: (starts to sob)

Th: (empathically) *What happened?*

R: *My father was always cold and aloof and forbid me to get emotional, to have feelings. So I would hide my feelings and never show them. He always made me feel shameful and dirty when I expressed any form of emotion.*

Th: *That is very helpful. So you are saying you come here already prescripted and preprogrammed not to show emotions. And you are proving to me that you can show them.*

R: *I couldn't help myself.*

Th: *But if you don't show emotions, then you will be nothing but a robot, and you will remain feeling paralyzed.*

R: *I do feel paralyzed.*

Th: *You say you feel paralyzed but you are not paralyzed. How you feel is not what you are in reality.*

R: *I am just not happy and I know I will never ever be happy.*

Th: *But happiness is not our goal now. Right now our job is to keep you functioning. To move at as slow a pace as you have to. Even if you have to crawl at a snail's pace to get up and dressed in the morning. At least you will be functioning.*

R: *What would you say if I said I don't want to function?*

Th: (the therapist addresses the language of dialectics) *Then I would say that isn't true because if it were true you wouldn't be here. But for someone not functioning, you are doing a great job giving me a sense of what the main issues are. I know you feel bad about abandoning your girlfriend. You do need to call her and face your feelings. Depression is an easy mask to hide under. We will continue next week. I am here if need be.*

Discussion

Rick's revelation made him realize his depression was a cover-up for fear of intimacy. At the root of his depression was the awareness that as bad as the depression made him feel at least it was "safer" than having to reveal his love and true self to his girlfriend. In the transference, the therapist helps him work through his distorted view of intimacy, dependency, and vulnerability so that he eventually realizes that withdrawal and disappearance from himself and the object world is what is "sick," and that his feelings and emotions are healthy. As therapy continued, Rick understood that he not only felt the pain, the loneliness, the isolation, and withdrawal, but he also became the pain. Patients who exhibit primitive defenses often cannot distinguish the difference between feeling the pain and becoming the pain. It is a very primitive state of mind. If a person feels cold, for instance, he can express the coldness with words. At more extreme levels of psychosis, the psychotic will *become* the cold (e.g., the frozen iceberg).

When one is clinically depressed, there's a very strong urge to pull away from others and to shut down. This is exactly the opposite of what is needed. Social isolation, withdrawal, and avoidance create more depression and exacerbate the condition. True clinical depression is a mood disorder in which feelings of sadness, loss, anger, or frustration interfere with everyday life for weeks or longer. Common elements can play a role in clinical depression. These include alcohol or drug abuse; medical conditions, including underactive thyroid, cancer, or long-term pain; certain medications such as steroids; and stressful life events.

Of all the types of disappearing males described so far, the borderline is perhaps the most lethal. At the onset borderlines come across as passionate and exciting. They will promise the world but because of the lack of impulse control, the false self, the inability to maintain object constancy they lose continuity. When threatened or betrayed, the depressed borderline male will lash out with a retaliatory response and self-mutilation, and will become the victim/self-sacrificial object. *Revenge my name is borderline!*

Borderlines often form pathological love bonds that have the tendency to repeat trauma again and again. This is known as traumatic bonding (Lachkar 2004b), where aggression and internal conflicts interfere with the capacity to maintain ongoing love bonds. Borderline depression occurs when these bonds have been depleted and the borderline has exhausted his reliable defenses and pretenses and no longer has the ego strength required to sustain what an intimate relationship requires. They bond with their objects through parasitic bonding, illness, and suicidal threats. Common symptoms of borderline depression and addiction include pervasive feelings of sadness, loneliness, and emptiness; general feelings of persecutory anxiety, feelings of hopelessness and desolation; poor use of transitional objects that causes the borderline to turn to addictive behaviors such as sexual addiction, drugs, gambling, alcohol, and drugs; restless, irritable thoughts of death or suicide; suicide attempts or plans.

I remember telling my borderline patient that I was going on vacation and would be away for two weeks, that I did have another therapist on call. However, if anything urgent came up I could always be contacted. The next day I get a call that he is planning to commit suicide. Instead of doing the usual routine—e.g., "Do you have a plan for how you would kill yourself?"—I first explored the possibility that this was his parasitic way of bonding with me and letting me know how he would miss me, needed me, because he could not express these feelings directly. I knew this was a bit risky, but knowing the patient felt persecuted by having needs and was terrified about feelings of dependency and vulnerability, I responded, "Steve, you don't need to threaten suicide to let me know how you will be feeling during our time of separation. Of course, you can commit physical suicide and end your life, but you can also commit emotional suicide, cutting off people from your life as you did with your girlfriend. She would have loved for you to express your feelings to her; instead, you attacked and threatened her when you began to feel close."

DEPRESSIVE POSITION

The depressive position is not to be confused with depressive disorders. According to Klein (1957), the paranoid-schizoid position is succeeded by the depressive position. The paranoid-schizoid position is a fragmented position in which thoughts and feelings are split off and projected because the psyche cannot tolerate feelings of pain, emptiness, loneliness, rejection, humiliation, or ambiguity. Klein viewed this position as the earliest phase of development, part-object functioning, and the beginning of the primitive superego (undeveloped).

In the depressive position, the person begins to perceive the other as a whole object (someone not only available for one's own self-serving purposes). It is a phase of development where there is a lessening of splitting and projective identification, hate, shame, blame, and attacking defenses; instead there is more room for ambivalence, tolerance, and desire to make reparation for one's wrongdoings. The depressive position is considered a healthy phase of development whereby the person begins to internalize his love objects, which leads to their restoration rather than destruction, as was prevalent in the paranoid position. The effort is toward coming to terms with guilt and the desire to restore the loved objects that were harmed.

The Case of Alan

Therapist: *Hi, Alan!*

Alan: *I feel so ashamed and embarrassed to even tell you what I've done.*

Th: *Well, you know you can tell me everything and anything.*

A: *I know I did wrong. I've been with my girlfriend for three years. I promised her the world, marriage, kids, a house. All along I knew it was a way of keeping her in the relationship. I knew if I told her that none of this was never going to happen she would leave me.*

Th: *So you betrayed her?*

A: *It is more than a betrayal. I devastated her when I called and told her I couldn't go on, that I was not prepared for marriage and that she was free to go on with her life.*

Th: *Do you love her?*

A: *Yes, but I felt stuck.*

Th: *So not knowing what to do, you just withdrew without making any effort to work things out with her.*

A: *I feel terrible, and I am very depressed.*

Th: *Actually, Alan, you are not depressed.*

A: *Then if I am not depressed, what am I?*

Th: *You are going through normal feelings of loss, and the fact that you feel sad and remorseful is a good sign.*

A: *Good to feel sad and so down on myself?*

Th: *Yes, you mishandled the situation and now you are experiencing feelings of guilt. You felt stuck, which means you had ambivalent feelings and didn't know how to handle them. I have a feeling you would like to repair the damage but are not sure how.*

A: *I do! I do want to very much. I feel terrible that I have hurt and betrayed her.*

Th: *Alan, you've just proved the point. You do not have a clinical depression. This is situational, and it can be repaired. You also have to know that even though you take all the responsibility for the false hopes and promises, your girlfriend also had an opportunity to make choices and could have moved on. Yet, this still does not absolve you from treating her badly.*

A: *I will call her.*

Th: *Good. I look forward to hearing more about it next week. See you then!*

Discussion

This case demonstrates how the therapist navigates the intermittent movement between the paranoid-schizoid position and the depressive position. Alan was clearly moving toward seeing his girlfriend as a whole object, one who has legitimate needs and whom he has betrayed. The therapist helps him contain the feelings of guilt and shame, while guiding him into the depressive position. At the same time, she leaves a small window of opportunity for him to see that this was not entirely his fault. The therapist's main effort was to confront his fears and help him understand that he was not experiencing a clinical depression, but was "transitioning" through normal states of sadness and loss. The prognosis in this case looks promising—a man who disappears and then reappears!

SUMMARY

Although there is considerable overlap, it is important to distinguish between the different kinds of depression: normal depression, depression caused by chemical imbalance, clinical or major depression. This chapter discusses these various levels of depression, including the depressive position as outlined by Melanie Klein. They demonstrate the disappearing male's proclivity to withdrawal and avoidance, obviously causing much pressure and consternation in their relations with women. Except for major depression, they all share in common omnipotent fantasies of entitlement and a preoccupation with the self to the exclusion of the needs and concerns of others. *I don't care if I kill myself. I will be free and you will be the ones to suffer!* The main task and challenge for the therapist is to continually remind the patient of reality and how the forces of splitting and projective identification, self-blame, and self-hatred deplete the ego's capacity to function and give way to a tendency to magnify and distort.

It is shocking and traumatic for a caretaker-type woman involved with a borderline depressive male to find that her lover has cut off all contact with her. He has either committed suicide, has been hospitalized, or is so withdrawn that he no longer has the capacity to maintain contact. This is devastating for the woman. It is important for the therapist to help this woman avoid identifying with the depressive's disappearance, to get through to her that she is not responsible.

Although we as therapists do not have crystal balls, we are often called on to answer the most commonly asked question from dumped women: "Do you think he will ever come back? Will he reappear?" Of course, we have no real answer. But what we can do is to offer some solace by letting the women know the most positive outcome involves the man who is in the depressive position, because this means he realizes his mistakes and wants very much to repair the damage he has caused—in which case therapy can help him salvage the relationship. In more severe cases it is questionable if the relationship can be put back together. The probability is not very good.

Chapter Nine

The Cross-Cultural Disappearing Male

Today our consultation rooms are packed with individuals and couples from various ethnic and cultural backgrounds. In many countries nationalism becomes the replacement for the American Dream. Therapists today face a new challenge with globalization. When people from different countries marry, they don't just marry a person; they tie a knot with another culture. How does a Western therapist deal with the various psychodynamics that present themselves with different cultural orientations? What intimacy or dependency means in one culture may have an entirely different meaning in another. Globalization and the war on terror have maximized our understanding of terrorism and malignant narcissistic leaders (Lachkar 2008a, 2008b) whose entitlement makes them think they can dominate the world. As a psychohistorian, I have found that people from third-world countries where there have been governmental and parental abuse, betrayal, and deprivation defend against shame by developing manic defenses to save face when they come to our country.

The focus of this chapter is mainly on Asia and the Middle East, whose cultures have contrasting dynamics to those of the West. In addition, these are countries in which women inherently take on a subordinate role to men. Islamic imperialism is not only a nationalistic threat; it has been a psychological war playing on people's fears and vulnerabilities. The disappearing male syndrome in the West takes on a completely different shape than in Asia and the Middle East. In the West men are programmed to show deference to the female, whereas Asian and Middle Eastern men reference an entire culture that has legitimated neglecting and abandoning their women.

Many researchers have referred to Middle Eastern and Asian societies as shame/honor cultures (Berton 2001; Lachkar 1997), as opposed to countries like Germany or France that can be characterized as having guilt cultures. In discussing culture, it is important to note that the way a Muslim man "disappears" is quite different than the way a Japanese man or even a Korean (or Chinese, Indonesian, Saudi Arabian, etc.) "disappears." For example, the Muslim will withdraw financial support and emotions, engage in polygamy, or stone and beat women if there is any suspicion of adultery or betrayal or if she has shamed or dishonored him. The Japanese male will withdraw or work even longer hours to avoid the female whom he believes has brought dishonor to him. Western culture supports and honors women and has laws that guarantee her human rights, as opposed to regimes where an entire culture has made her nonexistent.

Critics argue that men have not "disappeared" in the Asian and Muslim world because they were never there in the first place (Lachkar 2011). What "disappearance" means in the West often does not translate to diverse cultures. In *International Relations*, Professor Peter Berton (2001), a scholar on Japanese studies, gives the example of how the Japanese male is rarely present in the home and likens him to a 7-Eleven store: "Leaves at 7 a.m. and returns home at 11 p.m." At the more extreme level, the Islamic suicide bombers literally "disappear" after blowing themselves up as they "honor" their country and their families. Not only do these men disappear, but major historical episodes do, too. The Japanese are still denying their part in WWII war crimes, and Ahmadinejad to this day insists the Holocaust never took place.

The linkage is not only to physical or emotional disappearance, but to a cultural one as well. An entire culture can be prescripted to abandon and devalue its women. For example, it is important for psychologists and sociologists to note that Islamic culture follows the dictum of the Qur'an and Sharia Law, the Muslim constitution that controls every practice in the Muslim world. According to the standards of the West, these laws are abusive, traumatic, and in violation of human rights.

> *Allah has made men superior to women because men spend their wealth to support them. Therefore, virtuous women are obedient, and they are to guard their unseen parts as Allah has guarded them. As for women whom you fear will rebel, admonish them first, and then send them to a separate bed, and then BEAT them. But if they are obedient after that, then do nothing further; surely Allah is exalted and great!* (Qur'an 4:34)

One wonders how an entire society bonds and joins together in a collective group fantasy. To go against the group's customs, traditions, and ideology brings shame and humiliation to the group. Those who do not conform to these rules become enemies, outsiders, and are isolated from the group. Masao Miyamoto (1995) notes that the key concepts to understanding Japan's culture are narcissism and masochism. Although many have challenged the notion that Japan is "narcissistic," Miyamoto presents a critique of the "closed society" of the Japanese bureaucracy. This Tokyo-born psychiatrist refused to accept the formalized Japanese lifestyle. He ventured to question the bureaucracy and encountered a storm of criticism. Miyamoto's main concern was that Japan, despite its modern veneer and seemingly international flavor, is far behind other industrial nations in terms of lifestyle. He used his insight as a psychiatrist to show that avoidance of provoking envy, preservation of the status quo, and demonstrations of masochism provide the glue that holds this xenophobic system together. I refer to this as "reverse narcissism," whereby a group of people is dominated by the needs of the group and the culture rather than the omnipotent grandiose self.

Although I see Japan as having many narcissistic qualities, my view is that shame/blame cultures are more inclined toward borderline organization rather than narcissism. Being a group society rather than a "me–me" society attests to my collective diagnosis of Japan. Another example is offered by Kenneth Adams (2012), who unequivocally recognizes masochism as a primary element in Japanese culture. Children are used as scapegoats and helpless victims by absent fathers and suffocating mothers. Adams claims nothing has changed in Japanese society regarding the gender roles. Men are preprogrammed to sacrifice themselves to the workplace and women to the home and children. He notes that the Japanese male still shows devotion to the master and has an inherent warrior/sword mentality, albeit his identification has now shifted to the workplace. He refers to this as the "salary man" mentality, an archetype of the *Nihonjin* warrior—the same kind of aggression but translocated to a new generation.

In spite of its productive and economic growth, Japan still remains an institutionalized, masochistic, and sacrificial society. Economically, there has been a financial boom. Women are more active in the workplace, and the desire for home and marriage is of less importance. Even though Japanese men wear a different armor, they are still hard-wired to be warriors. On the surface it appears as though they have relinquished their undying loyalty to the master and have abandoned their swords, but basically the slavish devotion, self-sacrifice, and masochism still exist. Even though capable of pleasure and possessed of many opportunities, the masochist avoids or undermines pleasurable experiences. He still sacrifices his life for his boss and company and even to some extent for his wife and children. As the common wisdom of Japanese housewives goes, "*Teishu wa genki de rusu ga ii*," meaning "A good husband is healthy and absent."

CULTURAL RELATIVISM

Before describing the psychodynamics of the cultures we're addressing, it is essential to examine the cultural differences by taking into account the traditions, ideologies, values, treatment of women, and child-rearing practices—not so much as a defensive stance, but as something inherent in the culture. In today's expanding and ever-changing world, therapists, social workers, anthropologists, and governmental and judicial officials need to consider cross-cultural distinctions.

According to Endleman (1989), cross-culture means looking at culture from within, which attests to the notion that people who embody various traditions, ideologies, and religions are governed by certain psychological and cultural principles. Therefore, they do not share the same instinctual drives that others may have, and assume that universal laws regarding human development do not apply to them. Transculture views culture from without and assumes that all people are governed by the same universal laws regarding human needs and desire, and that men in every culture share the need to overcome oedipal rivals to be become masters of their own lives and fate. Endleman argues that Middle Eastern cultures are sadomasochistically enacting their hatred and envy toward women and are supported by governmental abuse (Lachkar 2011). *You cannot beat your wife here. That is considered abuse and you can get arrested for domestic violence. But in my country we are allowed to beat our wives when they are disobedient!*

The Islamic court system relegates women to a lower status. According to the Qur'an, a woman's testimony is worth only half that of a man. In cases of alleged rape, women are considered to be lying unless four male eyewitnesses testify to having seen the act occur. Being convicted of lying about rape carries punishments ranging from imprisonment and flogging to death by stoning. Acts such as stoning and honor killings are considered heroic. This is in keeping with a 7th-century edict issued by Muhammad. In our society we would diagnose this man as a sociopath, someone with no conscience or expression of remorse. Furthermore, property and inheritance rights of Muslim women are grossly unfair compared to those of men. Islamic law mandates that a son's inheritance should be twice the size of that of a daughter: "Allah [thus] directs you as regards your children's [inheritance]: to the male, a portion equal to that of two females" (4:11). We would think that in this modern era, Islamic courts would have evolved to seek more justice between men and women.

In the recent film *A Separation* (2012), filmmaker Asghar Farhadi goes beyond his cultural tradition to seek a balance more in keeping with a humanitarian approach (women in charge of money, man's dependency on women and his appreciation for women), and at the same time revealing the injustices toward women. The movie begins with an average couple in Tehran seemingly getting a divorce, then suddenly morphs into a nightmare of cultural horrors. The husband has to swallow his pride and beg his wife to return home as he struggles to accept her "newfound freedom." The filmmaker was walking a tightrope, well aware that he could veer only so far from the culture and still maintain credibility Even the Islamic judge aspired to show some fairness toward women while pointing out the injustices women faced (Highland 2012, personal communication). The positive aspect of the film is that the filmmaker shows that the desire for women's liberty and freedom does exist, and the influence of the West cannot be denied. He chose to show a modern-day Muslim wife leaving her husband of her own free will without repercussions. We see the "shame" as the husband struggles with his pride and the shame of having to depend on and need a woman.

CULTURAL INTERPLAY FROM EAST TO WEST

In today's world of multiculturalism, therapists continually encounter these contrasting dynamics. The line that separates culture and pathology is porous. Treating those from other cultures can be very bewildering, and therapists often feel overwhelmed, wondering how they can learn about all these dynamics. What is considered abuse in our country is considered "normal" in another. Emotional and physical abuse has many roots in cultures where women are taught that true love means that you please your man and care for him even at the sacrifice of the self (more prevalent in Asian and Middle Eastern than Western societies). Many women feel equally abused when their husbands show deference to parents and thus emotionally abandon or dismiss their wives.

First, let us focus on the junction between culture and psychopathology. Western mental health professionals continue to struggle with helping people—especially women from shame/honor cultures—find a sense of self or self-identity. The women in these cultures are continuously trying to get their society to see them as separate and autonomous individuals. In many societies the focus on the self is virtually nonexistent. Those in the West belong to what we consider to be an individualistic culture (an "I/me" society), where emphasis is on self-development. In Asian and Middle Eastern societies the emphasis is on the group self or the collective group self. American culture places emphasis on uniqueness and self-expression, whereas Asian societies lean heavily on the ideology of the group and community, society, or nation. So when we talk about a self, are we talking about an individual self? A group self? A self-actualized self? Or a collective group self?

For most mental health professionals, just being aware that there are differences across cultures can be helpful. Dependency, shame, honor, and peace have different meanings in different cultures. It is not enough to understand shame without understanding the need to "save face." Even words like "opportunity" and "honor" can be poles apart. In the West we associate the term "opportunity" with man's freedom to flourish. In the Muslim world "opportunity" could mean the permission to stone, slaughter, or even behead a woman who exposes her arms or face or goes out in public unaccompanied. The same holds true for terms such as "honor" and "peace." In Islamic regimes, only when all the infidels are destroyed can there be peace and harmony.

For the Japanese, peace or "*wa*" means the desire to be at one with others, devoid of conflict, envy, and confrontation. In Japan, dependency is inextricably linked to the concept of *amae*, the relationships between the mother and infant and her ability to read her baby's mind without him ever having to ask for anything (Doi 1973; Berton 1995; Lachkar 2008, 2011). To maintain these positions, the Japanese have two selves—the true and false self, *honne* and *tatamae* (Berton 1995; Lachkar 2008, 2011). Therapists also need to be aware of the hierarchical positions whereby deference to country, elders, big brother, and boss come first and wives and children are last on the list. For example, Zhou Yan, a Chinese Olympic Gold Medal skater champion in 2000, was criticized for thanking her parents first and not her country. The same holds true for other Chinese athletes, such as basketball sensation Jeremy Lin, whose skill at basketball is not considered as his own personal accomplishment, but as giving honor to his country (Kaiman 2012).

In contrast to most Asian women (culturally speaking of course), who are rather submissive, Korean women have become more aggressive for they are the only ones who were abandoned by their men through no fault of their own. Hordes of Korean men were killed during WWII, leaving many wives and children without husbands and fathers. Korean women had to learn to fend for themselves, and they became very bitter and rageful, known in Korean as "*han*." This term has deep historical significance (Lachkar 2008, 2011).

> *I cannot think of any need in childhood as strong as the need for a father's protection.*
>
> Sigmund Freud, *Civilization and Its Discontents*

Many have referred to Japan as being xenophobic, unwilling to allow foreigners to enter Japanese society despite outwardly seeming to be hospitable. By comparison, the Islamists are extremists. They will not only allow foreigner" infidels" to enter, they are likely to kill or behead them. Because of their lack of identity with strong male role models and their mothers, who are virtually nonexistent, Islamic men identify with aggressive, powerful leaders like terrorists who become the fantasized savior fathers who take them to Paradise. Vaknin (2007) refers to this as the most severe form of malignant narcissism or masochistic love—which is when a person is prone to self-defeating, punishing, self-destructive behaviors. Not having the role models to help overcome and master their oedipal rivals developmentally, how could they be available to women? As much as they need them, they must destroy them.

It is always puzzling how people are mesmerized by and revere leaders who starve, abuse, and mistreat their people—sadistic and cruel dictators like Slobodan Milosevic, Saddam Hussein, Arafat, Kadafi, Hitler, Stalin. These malignant personalities offer a dream, a fantasy that they can achieve something better. Hitler for example, offered a purer, cleaner, more sterile country without the contamination of the "dirty Jews." In short, these men all served as "father figures." As cruel and sadistic as these leaders are, they constitute a presence and provide reassurance for the fatherless male. Islam culture has many orphans and abandoned children. In fact, it is astonishing how many leaders in the Middle East, ranging from Ishmael to the prophet Mohammed, were orphaned and abandoned. Asia, a shame society in which overt expression is forbidden and people must hide their needs and desires, may have revered Kim because he was able to exploit his wealth and power shamelessly. This could make quite an impact on a group of repressed people. *If I can do it, you can, too!*

THE CROSS-CULTURAL V-SPOT

Is there such a thing as a "cultural V-spot?" Do nations, countries, and societies have a V-spot, whereby an entire culture adheres to certain group fantasies based on painful archaic injuries, myths, and sentiments handed down from generation to generation. Yes, I believe they do! The noted psychoanalyst Carl Jung (1973) referred to this as the collective group consciousness. This could be a biblical or historical past, a group genocide, a holocaust—something that evokes painful, injurious feelings and old memories. The cultural V-spot is a collective group fantasy, an area of vulnerability traumatically bonded through wars, loss, or a lifetime of governmental violations of human rights abuse that keeps a group embroiled in endless feuds. This traumatic bonding with an archaic injury never reaches conflict resolution. It is what James Grotstein (1981) refers to as the black hole, the never-ending search for identity, a search for meaning in the meaninglessness. There are striking parallels between marital and political conflict. It seems that entire cultures and nations, like couples, can engage in ongoing, painful, destructive interactions without ever reaching any conflict resolution.

Therapists today need to ask: Where do culture and pathology meet? One culture's mental health is another culture's pathology. Some say terrorists or jihadists are normal people who merely have been brainwashed to fight for a cause. One man's terrorist is another man's freedom fighter. But according to Western psychological studies and standards of human development, they are not normal. To penetrate these seemingly impermeable borders, we must take into account certain aspects of culture such as (1) childrearing practices, ideology, mythology and (2) psychodynamics of shame, guilt, envy, jealousy, control/domination, and dependency; and we must try to determine how these collective traumas are qualitatively and culturally experienced.

It is noteworthy that third-world countries rarely have clinical programs devoted to human development and human research. Many are already preordained to condone the mistreatment and violation of women, behavior that is justified based on tradition and religion. The most striking aspect of the cultural V-spot is its lack of fairness and its impact on the treatment of women: men can mistreat women, but women cannot mistreat men.

TREATMENT POINTS AND TECHNIQUES

Following are the main elements that the therapist should keep in mind when dealing with the disappearing cross-cultural male:

- Understand the fundamental differences in the dynamics of the cultures involved.
- Empathize with the resistances and the differences but *not* with the aggression.
- Self-psychology and mirroring are most effective in reflecting the aggression.
- Try to locate the cross-cultural hook to find pathology within the cultures involved.
- Remind the couple why they came to you in the first place.
- Set treatment goals.
- Be familiar with the basics of the culture—e.g., the music, the foods, a few expressions, greetings.
- Make use of the language of empathology and the language of dialectics.
- Be aware of body language and position (sitting too close, shaking hands, etc.).
- Focus less on the cure and more on acceptance and tolerance of cultural differences.
- Remember that all therapists are mandated reporters, and abuse and violations must be reported regardless of what another culture dictates.
- Use humor to avoid sounding punitive or hooking into shame or guilt.

In exploring cross-culture, I devised the concept of the cross-cultural hook as a means to find pathology within one's own culture (Lachkar 2008b). This technique pinpoints pathology by spotting contradictions or hypocrisy within one's own culture. For example, a Japanese wife finds solace in nursing her baby while sleeping with the baby in another room. She states that this is a common practice in her culture. The therapist then has an opportunity to point out the conflict with Western culture. Another example is an American wife married to a Japanese man who complains that he is cheap, and does not believe in our materialistic society. In reality, it is quite the opposite: Japan happens to be a hub of materialism, and invests a great deal in shopping and of course, technology. In fact, objects often become the replacement for human contact.

Treating individuals or couples from another culture can be overwhelming and cause much frustration, not only because therapists may not have an understanding of their languages, traditions, childrearing practices, or identities, but because some of the resistance and rigidity to adapt to their current environment is so embedded in these patients. The following is an example of an American woman who was married to a Muslim man.

He always left me behind, as if I didn't exist. I never knew where he went. He never invited me to family events, parties, celebrations; he took our son and daughter, but not me. He had numerous affairs, and when I threatened to divorce him he told me he would leave me with no money and take our children away from me. And that's what happened when I finally did divorce him. The judge in his homeland granted sole custody to my husband. He accused me of being an unfit mother, and the judge supported him. She said my duty was to "obey"!

Aggression toward women is bound to cause transference issues. Dealing with transference, countertransference, and couples transference becomes quite a challenge for Western therapists. Many therapists are seduced by the rhetoric that the aggression and violations against women are culturally induced. What follows are some examples of the complications that can occur when dealing with individuals from countries that sanction abuse and mistreatment of women.

- Therapist overempathizes with the aggressor.
- Therapist may feel the aggressor is entitled to his right to violate women because it is culturally based.
- Therapist may not be culturally sensitive or informed.
- Therapist may be frightened of the aggressor and feels she must conform.
- Therapist may so angry with the aggressor that she may overreact.
- Therapist must find a way to segue into "the couple transference."

The Case of Marcia and Amir

Amir, who is from Iraq, has been married for three years to an American woman. They have a two-year-old child. The therapist attempts to open up the therapeutic space through the couple transference. During treatment, their case presented the issue of hierarchy between the mother-in-law and the wife.

Theapist: *Salam* (therapist greets the couple in Arabic and starts to shake hands, but notices that Amir pulls his hand away and shows no eye contact).

Amir: *Salam* (hello).

Th: *Please have a seat, and we shall begin. So, I would like to hear from each of you. Who would like to start?*

Marcia: *I will start.*

A: *No, I will start.*

Th: *Very well.*

A: *My wife does not understand that in our culture women must show obedience to their husbands. She must understand that when my mother invites me I must go, but she gets upset when she remains at home.*

M: *Upset isn't the word. I go ballistic! Who goes to a party or an event and does not include their wife or child?*

A: *My first allegiance is to my mother, and in my country the wife understands this. I have been trying to explain this to her, but she doesn't get it.*

Th: *But things are different in our country. Here men treat their women with respect and as equals.*

A: *I understand that. But Marcia knew this when she married me.*

M: *No, I certainly did not! How did I know that when I did not "obey" your commands you would beat me and hit me?*

Th: *Is this true?*

A: *Yes, that is my right. And you know what she did? She called the police.*

Th: *And what did they do?*

A: *They put me in a class with a bunch of sissy boys to teach us anger management. What they don't understand is it is not anger. It is our right as men.* (starts to recite the Qur'an) *Allah says admonish them first, and then beat them.*

Th: *So you feel it is your right to beat your wife?*

A: *Not only is it my right, it is my duty.*

Th: *Your "duty" can put you in prison.*

M: *See what I have to live with?*

Th: *Yes, and this is why you are both here. Amir, I am impressed that you would choose an American therapist, and a Jewish one at that! There must be some part of you that does want to adapt to our way of life* (opening up the couple transference and the cross-cultural hook).

M: *Good point. Why would he choose you or me?*

Th: *Yes, Amir, you could have married a Muslim woman and chosen a Muslim therapist.*

A: *I happen to like American women. I find them very attractive and sexy.*

M: *You should see his porno sites.*

Th: *Yes, and as much as you find "us" attractive" and lust after us, you must destroy us, because you cannot allow yourself to need us or be dependent.*

A: (looking toward Marcia) *What is she talking about?*

M: *She is right. You cannot allow yourself to be needy or to depend upon women as nurturers. You can only depend on your mother! He acts like a true and faithful Muslim, but he steps out of his tradition when it suits him. Even in his own country he would drink, not pray, eat pork. Yet when it comes to me he suddenly becomes a devout Muslim* (therapist didn't have to find the cross-cultural hook; Marcia did it for her).

Th: *Marcia, you are finding contradictions in Amir's behavior?*

A: *Hold on! I did not come here for you to shame or dishonor me.*

Th: *What you call shame, I find very healthy because it helps me understand that behind your "traditional" flag is a very healthy, normal man who would like to be freer to express himself, to love, to be vulnerable. I think you both did an excellent job in helping me understand not only your cultural differences, but how underneath all this are two people with real and legitimate needs. Can we meet next week at this time?*

A: *I guess so. As long as you wear a burka.*

Th: (laughs) *I see you have not lost your sense of humor.*

M: *Great! See you then.*

A: (looking therapist in the eye) *Salam!*

Th: *Salam!*

Discussion

In this case the therapist uses the language of dialectics to show the conflicts between the couple's real needs—how under the guise of religion Amir hides his dependency needs and vulnerabilities (can rely on his mother but not his American wife), how he chooses an American wife and an American therapist, and how he "loves" us and yet rejects us. The therapist uses the cross-cultural hook to show empathy with the difficulty of adapting and adjusting to another culture. The therapist had to curtail her own countertransference issues: her rage toward him when he said it was okay to be abusive to his wife. She tried her best to let him know that in our country it is a criminal offense and he could go to jail, even though in his country it was acceptable. Mirroring the conflicts and the using the language of empathology were most effective in this case. The therapist cautiously offered sympathy about the difficulty of adaptation but not toward the aggression. Cultural traditions and religious laws can never be a rationale for abuse, violence, and the mistreatment of women.

The case that follows shows how the therapist attempts to mirror the couple's cultural differences while at the same time pointing out the contradictions, using many of the techniques mentioned above. Yoshi really never wanted to leave Japan, his work, his boss, or his family. He succumbed to the wishes of his wife, Beth, and moved to America because he could not tolerate the shame of a divorce. Meanwhile, Beth has difficulty understanding and accepting her husband's inability to adapt to an American lifestyle. Yoshi now has more time and freedom, which Beth believes he should be spending at home with family.

The Case of Yoshi and Beth

Beth: *It's horrible. The children and I hardly ever see Yoshi.*

Therapist: *Oh, why is that?*

B: *Because Yoshi is always away at night, while I am home with the kids.*

Th: *This must make you feel very alone, especially when you desire to be intimate with your husband.*

B: *Well, who wouldn't want their husband home at night instead of out drinking sake with the guys?*

Yoshi: (in a very soft-spoken tone) *You see, in Tokyo it is quite common for the woman to stay home and take care of the home and the children. We men work long hours, and at the end of the day we need to relax.*

B: *But this is not Tokyo! Why can't you relax with me? Why do you need to get hot baths and massages?*

Th: *Sounds as though you are very angry.*

B: *Anger isn't the word. I am actually beginning to resent our kids.*

Y: (again in a soft-spoken voice) *Beth doesn't understand. Japanese men are devoted to their work. We form a very special relationship with our boss and our work.*

Th: *But this is not what we do in this country. In this country the children feel abandoned if the father is not present. You are also making your wife and children feel ousted from society because they are unlike other wives and children whose husbands and fathers are present. In your country the wife and children are proud to have a father hard at work* (therapist mirroring the cultural difference and throwing in a cross-cultural hook).

Y: *I understand that, but it is hard to get over a custom that has existed for thousands of years.*

B: *This is what I get all the time!*

Th: *Yes, it is hard. Nevertheless, Yoshi, you were able to break away from your culture when you chose to marry an American woman, a Westerner.*

Y: *This is true. But she also married me, a Japanese man, and this is the way it is.*

Th: Actually, *it really isn't, because in your country men work from 7 a.m. to 11 p.m., even on weekends, and hardly take vacations. Here we have certain hours, and your organization opens at 9 a.m. and closes at 5 p.m. It is even closed for holidays, so you do have time to spend with your wife and family. So now you need to acquiesce to your wife's desire, maybe give her some* amae (the cross-cultural hook).

B: *The needs of women are recognized in America.*

Th: *Yoshi, I hope you appreciate that in our country you can have the best of both worlds: the freedom to work and time to play.*

B: *In our country he would be shamed for ignoring his wife and family.*

Th: *Beth is making a good point. In your country you would be shamed for staying home and making cupcakes, but in our country you would be shamed for abandoning your wife and child. It would be as if I went to Japan and returned my food to a waiter because the fish wasn't cooked enough.*

B: *That's really a good example, but Yoshi simply disappears and has no shame.*

Th: *Beth, with all due respect, you need to be a little patient. Yoshi has been here for less than a year and it does take time to adapt. Yet, I can tell you really love your wife* (Yoshi blushes).

B: *Yoshi has a very hard time with feelings. He feels ashamed to admit that he loves me and the kids.*

Th: *Yoshi, one way to avoid feelings is to work. When you work you can hide, because in your country feelings are shameful. But we can deal with this another time. Meanwhile, it will take time to get accustomed to having the freedom for pleasure and happiness that this country offers you. Shall we meet again next week?*

Y: *I can't. I have to work.*

Th: *Now you are disappearing on me. And if you do, there won't be a me here to help you, which is why I believe you are here in the first place* (couple transference). *Yet, I am very impressed that you are here because in Japan this would be frowned upon.*

Y: (laughs) *You shamed me into it.*

Th: *Sayonara!*

Y: *Sayonara!*

Discussion

Yoshi appears to be genuinely attached to his culture, but, actually, he hides his true feelings and dependency needs under his devotion to tradition and his job. As the case unfolds, we begin to see how preprogrammed he is to be the dutiful employee, devoted to his boss and master. The therapist applies the cultural hook and mirroring techniques by showing Yoshi how he is not giving his wife *amae* or paying attention to what she needs. In addition, the therapist helps him realize that he is shamefully mistreating his wife and children by being an absent husband and father. She also shows that his work does not warrant obsessively long hours. The therapist uses a great deal of mirroring to reflect sympathy and sensitivity to each partner while highlighting the dynamics operative within both their diverse worlds.

Many Japanese women today are marrying Americans because they are frustrated by having to stay home and take care of finances and children while their husbands work long and tedious hours, even when they're not in Japan. In treatment the therapist must be very cautious not to shame or humiliate the Japanese man but rather to bond with him and embrace his culture by mirroring his experience. *It is nice for families to have time to do things together. Working long hours and going out later is typical in Japan, but here husbands are more involved with their children. In your culture you are revered for being devoted to your work and to your boss.* At this point the therapist can throw in her cross-cultural hook: *It is difficult to adapt to the differences. It would be as if I went to Japan and didn't bow, or went to a conference and sat with the men, and then said, "Well, in our country we don't bow and we don't separate the men from the women."*

Yodo and Alfred: The Case of the Nursing Mother

Alfred: *I can't stand it anymore. We hardly have sex.*

Therapist: *And why is that?*

A: *Because Yodo is always nursing our son.*

Th: *Nursing is a normal part of life. Why would it interfere with your ability to be intimate?*

A: *Because our son is five years old.*

Th: *Oh, I see. Way beyond the weaning years.*

A: *You bet. Every time I go into the bedroom there is Yodo watching TV, and Yoshi is just sucking away.*

Th: *You sound very angry.*

A: *I am. I'm also beginning to resent our son.*

Yodo: (softly) *Alfred doesn't understand. Japanese mothers nurse their babies, especially their sons, until around five or so. This way we form a special relationship between mother and son.*

Th: *But this is not what we do in this country.*

Y: *I understand. But this custom has existed for centuries. It makes me a good mother.*

A: *See what I'm talking about?*

Th: *But you did break away from your culture when you chose to marry a Westerner.*

Y: *Yes, but I am a Japanese woman, and this is our culture.*

Th: *Actually, it really isn't, because if you were to follow the customs in your culture, the woman would acquiesce to the man's desires* (the cross-cultural hook).

Y: *Here women are free to do what they need to do. I think this is what I love about this country. Men treat women with respect.*

Th: *Yodo, so here you have the best of both worlds: the freedom to nurse your son as you please and be respected and treated with equality. But you are insensitive to your husband's needs.*

Y: *In my country we give each other* amae, *a certain way without words, showing the other what we really need.*

Th: *I respect and appreciate that, but as the therapist here I have to show* amae *to both of you. What happens to your* amae *when you are not in harmony (*wa*) with your husband's need for intimacy? If you are telling us how important it is, then where is your* amae*?*

Y: (puts her head down in shame)

Th: *Yodo, I do not mean to shame or humiliate you. In fact, I very much appreciate the beauty and wonderful traditions your country brings us. I am trying to help you understand your husband's needs and let you know that in this country nursing usually ends by the first year or so.*

Y: *I guess I am hiding my true feelings (*hone*) because I am really afraid if I let go of my son, I will have nothing because my husband will run off.*

Th: *You mean as the men in Japan do: work long hours, go to Geisha houses, and abandon the wife and children?*

Y: (sobbing)

A: *Yodo, no, that won't happen. I love you. In fact, it is the opposite. I want to be with you.*

Th: *What a blessing and joining of two cultures right before my very eyes. Yodo, I know it is hard to express feelings because it is often considered a sign of weakness in your culture. In our country it is a sign of strength.*

A: *Thank you, doctor.*

Th: *See you next week.*

Discussion

While Yodo appears to be attached to her culture, she is hiding her true feelings behind the Japanese banner. Her attachment to her son is not so much cultural as a defense against annihilation or abandonment anxiety, the fear that her husband will dismiss her and abandon her like a Japanese husband. In reality, Yoko was projecting this fantasy onto her husband because Alfred was not at all the "typical" workaholic, neglectful Japanese daddy/husband. In fact, quite the contrary, he was asking for more closeness and intimacy. Issues around shame, the role of women, and the true self were an integral part of this case. The cross-cultural hook was a technique to show Yodo how the very person who expects *amae* is the one who refrains from giving it. This highlights the cross-cultural narcissist, who expects to have everything from both worlds.

I am reminded again how essential it is to examine the cultural ramifications of the disappearing male, taking into account the traditions, ideology, values, treatment of women, and child-rearing practices. Where is the juncture between culture and pathology? Many therapists view the dynamics from other cultures as an upside-down world, a Mad Hatter's tea party. When we talk about disappearance, whose "disappearance" are talking about? When we talk about abuse, betrayal, withdrawal, isolation, whose kind of abuse are we referring to? Our disappearing male is different than the disappearing man in the Muslim world. Ours is based on psychological distinctions and defense mechanisms, and theirs is based on a doctrine designed to dictate man's behavior toward women. For example, the way a schizoid "disappears" when feeling suffocated is different than a narcissist who withdraws when narcissistically injured or an obsessive-compulsive when feeling endangered by dirt," or the passive-aggressive who projects his baby self into his partner, leaving all the responsibility up to the woman.

SUMMARY

Therapists cannot ignore the cultural, ethical, and religious aspects involved in treating people from various ethnic backgrounds. When people come to this country, the laws in their countries do not apply, and they are subject to the same rules as men in Western countries—as well as the same punishments for engaging in abuse and domestic violence. Treating male aggression and abuse of women and children under the guise of culture, religion, and tradition brings up many challenges for therapists trained in Western societies. In this chapter I have chosen to focus on two diverse cultures, Japan and Islam. Even though they are far apart, they both have contrasting dynamics to cultures that adhere to Judeo-Christian beliefs and Western laws.

There are complex and conflicting psychodynamics involved in treating cross-cultural issues. They include: shame vs. guilt, jealousy vs. envy, true self vs. false self, separation vs. fusion, group self vs. the individual self, pleasure vs. self-sacrifice and victimization, loyalty to family vs. loyalty to country vs. loyalty to elders/bosses/leaders, reality vs. magical thinking. The therapist must go beyond culture to see the universality of the human condition. It is not really about women, sex, religion, or tradition, but more about control, domination, submission, hatred, envy, and unresolved oedipal issues. The men in societies that perpetuate this way of thinking have not only "disappeared," but the women have been abandoned by an entire culture.

Chapter Ten

The Disappearing Woman

When I am with my boyfriend I feel fine, I feel whole, I feel content. But the moment he lays eyes on another woman, I don't know what happens to me. I feel as though I no longer exist. I know he is not interested in other women and this whole thing exists in my head. But now I am at the point when we go out, like to a restaurant, the first thing I do is case the place. I look around to see if there are attractive women and then try and get a table so that he is not facing one. I am contemplating getting plastic surgery so I can look like some of the women he glances at that I think he finds sexy and attractive. I have small boobs, so I will definitely get a boob job.

It follows that any attempt to comprehend and define the syndrome of the disappearing woman is not clear and concise. Analysis requires special attention to multiple factors. These include assessment of the disappearing woman in general terms, as a separate entity apart from her relationship, as well as within the context of her relationship. Another facet to be considered involves the economic and cultural expectations and demands bearing on her role in society. Finally, the woman's mental status within the realm of a personality disorder requires examination.

Within this framework I consider two general types of disappearing women. The most common and most widespread in clinical practice are the women that exhibit borderline organization, which includes the histrionic, the dependent, and the dissociative. These are the needy ones, the ones in constant search of an identity, the ones who define themselves solely in terms of their relationships, who lack object constancy, self-esteem, and make constant demands for reassurance. They are the naggers, the whiners, the complainers, those who bond via pain and engage is self-destructive, sabotaging behaviors. The histrionic is similar to the robotic male in that neither disappears physically; rather, they disappear emotionally and psychologically. Moreover, the histrionic disappears from her own needs, her own body, and from her own identity. An indication of even a hint of abandonment, jealousy, or threat of desertion, and she vanishes. *When he loves me I feel I exist; when he is mad or upset with me, I no longer exist.*

The second most common type of disappearing woman is becoming even more common. This is the "independent" woman who feels she no longer needs men. These women have become so tainted, jaded, and bitter that they develop an emotional armor that shouts their intention to the world: "Never again!" Within this continuum are women who are preprogrammed to fend and care for themselves without a man. An illustration of this is in vitro fertilization. *I don't need a father for my child. All I need is his sperm!* In addition, there is a certain segment of women so enraged with men that they not only resent men but are out to exact revenge from them. *They used me; now it's my turn to use them, Screw them all!*

We rented a lovely country home overlooking the ocean. Finally we were together—living in absolute bliss. It wasn't easy leaving a wife of 20 years and three kids, but I decided after working all these years as a busy architect and responding to everyone's demands that it was time for me to enjoy life. When I met Betty, I knew she was the woman of my dreams. Being an artist herself, she appreciated my fine taste in art and in furnishings. We ordered beautiful designer furniture, and every weekend we would go to art galleries to pick out sculptures and paintings. She was sexy as hell. I couldn't keep my hands off her. Unlike with my wife, whom I dreaded coming home to because there was the same monotonous conversation and activities, I would get an adrenalin rush with Betty. As tired as I was after work, I would drag her into the bedroom and would screw her brains off. Then came the shock. One day I rushed home to be with Betty, opened the door to our home, and guess what? Everything was gone. All the furniture, all the paintings, the art. Even the closet was bare. I was mortified. I did not know what to do so I called the police, but to no avail. They couldn't do anything. I am so mad at myself. I should have known. Betty repeatedly told me how she felt abused by men and couldn't trust them. She ran out on her last husband without a word and sent him divorce papers. I should have known better. I was such a fool.

Achieving an adequate assessment of the disappearing woman is complex, even after excluding the psychological, social, and cultural factors. These women do not live in a vacuum. They are the product of an ever-changing society. In the Introduction to this book, I mentioned that the breakdown of the family structure was due in part to the powerful forces of social change that are affecting all facets of the family. Modern society and urban living have placed the woman in an compromising position. She is under constant pressure to perform, achieve, and accomplish vis-à-vis her male counterparts, and to maintain a career while caring for a family. This plays out as the dialectic need to be loved countered by the need for independence, the ability to survive without men. This attitude was undreamt of a few decades ago. These generalizations have become increasingly evident in clinical practice. Henry Dicks (1967) punctuates the trend of the "new positive woman," remarking that the majority of families are exclusively "female made" (p. 19) and that the emancipation of women after the Second World War has had a dramatic impact on middle-class and working-class women. He concludes that a majority of these women have betrayed and defied their own biological, constitutional, and maternal capacities in order to be assimilated into a male-dominated culture that has devalued them.

Let us begin our exploration of the disappearing woman with the histrionic.

THE HISTRIONIC DISAPPEARING WOMAN

The histrionic is characterized by self-dramatization, an excessive need for attention, and an exaggerated display of emotion. She is exhibitionistic, seductive, overtly provocative, and displays other forms of inappropriate behaviors. She gets acutely anxious when not the center of attention, has a poor sense of reality testing and judgment, and imagines that men's interest in her is greater than it really is. Women with histrionic personality disorder often lack impulse control, throw temper tantrums, laugh loudly, and cry at the drop of a hat. The most common characteristics within this pathological disorder are exhibited by women with infantile and borderline personalities (a false self, a split self, a disassociated self). Marilyn Monroe's legacy as an American sex icon lives on after her death over 50 years ago because people still remain fixated on how such a glamorous movie star suffered so much and ended up dying so tragically. She had many personas, ranging from glamour queen to housewife, shy and innocent, intellectual, serious actress, and "dumb blond." As she told a close friend, "I've got many quivers to my bow. I can become anyone they want me to be" (Banner 2012). Her variety of husbands even provided extra credibility and further justification to enact these various personas.

Husband: *Every time I even look at another woman or give a woman a hug, she goes ballistic.*

Wife: *It is more than a hug. You kiss and squeeze them tightly.*

H: *I don't think that's what I do. You just overreact and get jealous.*

W: *Of course, I get jealous. Why you don't act that way with me?*

H: *I do! But when I do you push me away and tell me that I am just doing it because I feel guilty.*

W: *You should feel guilty. You have been neglecting me for a long time.*

H: *Well, maybe I have been neglecting you because you act insecure and overreact to everything I do.* (to therapist) *Why can't she just be a real woman? Why does she always have to put on such a show? Every little thing throws her. If she breaks a fingernail, she has a fit! It is as though she has disappeared from her body and is just a walking breast and vagina.*

W: (yelling) *I have a right to overreact when you give attention to other women and ignore me. Look what happened last night at the party—hugging every woman you saw.*

H: *Stop it! I can't take your constant accusations. I love you and that's all that counts.*

W: *You don't love me. If you loved me, you would give me more attention.*

H: *Your insecurity turns me off.*

Th: *So what do you do when you get turned off?*

H: *I just leave to get away from her nagging and go out with buddies and have a couple of beers.*

The disappearing histrionic woman is easily upset by any event that she finds even remotely perturbing and will react way out of proportion. Her very essence is about the continual need for approval and reassurance. Basically, her unavailability transfers to her partners, and her relations with men are short lived. *How do I look? What should I wear? Are you sure it looks okay?* Her anger and rage and other enactments become disproportionate to the "offense." Excessive parasitic dependency needs are exhibited with almost child-like naiveté.

These characteristics were most beautifully depicted in a 2011 film, *The Dangerous Method.* The movie tells the story of Freud and Jung treating a mutual patient, Sabrina Spielrein. Sabrina is the theatrical, histrionic patient who seduces Jung, while Freud riddles Jung with guilt. In another film, *My Week with Marilyn* (2011), we see a similar dynamic with the unstoppably seductive nature of Marilyn (it is very tempting to categorize this as the

"Marilyn Monroe Syndrome"!) focusing her wiles on a 23-year-old man who was working on the film she was making. The following vignette illustrates various features operative within this syndrome.

The Case of Sandy

Sandy is a 63-year-old woman, but looks fortyish. She came to therapy for assessment of a relational issue with her boyfriend. Sandy appeared in session wearing very high stiletto heels with a leopard skin body suit, tons of make-up, and lots of glitz. Sandy was very proud of herself. She is a vegan and works out daily with a trainer, and if she ever sees anyone in a cafe or restaurant eating meat, she does not hesitate for a moment to go over and scold them. She says she is only attracted to younger men, that the thought of being with a man who is her peer is unthinkable. "I don't want to be with those old men who can't even get it up. I look young, and many men are attracted to me."

She began to sob when expressing how completely devastated she felt when Bill, her latest boyfriend, broke up with her, saying he wanted to be with a younger woman. "This is when I lost it. I completely got out of control. I yelled and screamed and said, 'How dare you want to be with a younger woman? Are you saying I am not good enough for you?' He kept insisting that our relationship was over, that I was phony, did not act my age, was immature, and that I overreacted to the slightest provocation. I don't know what came over me and am surprised he didn't call the police. I started to throw things at him and began to hit him violently. He complained that I was overly emotional, too concerned with how I look, that I basically cared more about myself then him."

Sandy continued to cry hysterically, and there was nothing much I could say to console her. Finally, I mentioned that the breakup perhaps did not have so much to do with age but that it was more about a problem that emanated from her childhood—the need for excessive attention and how this need gets in the way of maintaining a healthy and caring relationship. Sandy showed a few moments of relief but then again began to cry hysterically. As much as I tried to reassure her, she continued to go on about how she knows she is better looking than most women, and that it is rare for women her age to do the kind of marathon working out she does.

Discussion

Sandy is the quintessential histrionic, with many narcissistic and borderline features. However, unlike the narcissist she does not withdraw; instead, she becomes violent, abusive, over-reactive and out of control. Again, unlike the narcissist, who tends to withdraw, Sandy does what many histrionic patients do: she disappears from her mind and a reality that she has long ago abandoned. Her body and sexuality constitute her only venue to human relations, and she uses them to enrapture or entice men. It seems curious how someone like Sandy, who is so clingy and needy, can "disappear." The first argument is that the term "disappear" is used interchangeably with splitting and disassociation. In addition, not only does the object become "unavailable," the histrionic becomes "unavailable" to herself. To clarify, I turn to Donald Meltzer's (1967) formulation that introduces us to the concept of psychic zones—how one person can emotionally and psychologically "live" within the mental space of the other. In my previous publications (Lachkar 2004b, 2008a, 2008b, 2009, 2011), I refer to this model frequently, showing how couples in the paranoid-schizoid position vanish from their own mental state and "live inside" the object. I find this relevant to the disappearing woman, how she splits off or abandons her own psychic state to virtually live inside the mental space of the other, akin to the "black hole." *If you love me I* exist; *if you don't love me or if you look at another woman, I vanish into nothingness.*

There are many variations of the histrionic woman that carry over to other personality disorders, including narcissistic, borderline, and obsessive-compulsive behaviors: narcissists because of their excessive entitlement, borderlines because of their lack of impulse control and uncontrollable rage, and obsessive-compulsives because of the high maintenance needed to keep one's body forever young and beautiful. Typically, the histrionic is very sexually manipulative and exhibits inappropriate behaviors; she is magnificently skilled in the art of alluring men. She is excessively needy, demanding, dependent, and, among other narcissistic qualities, displays a need for "all the attention."

Another type of histrionic woman goes to the opposite extreme and is preoccupied with psychosomatic illness. She doesn't really care much about how she looks or what she wears or her sexuality. Rather, she is more concerned with bonding with the pain and getting emotional gratification via devotion to her illness. Any hint of dirt or contamination can send her over the top. Although she may share many characteristics with the obsessive-compulsive, she is too needy and dependent to be confused with one.

The following case illustrates this aspect of the histrionic woman—achieving attention through psychosomatic symptoms. The conundrum these women present in treatment is how much is biological and how much is psychological, and where do these meet? It is always a therapeutic challenge to discern how to treat patients with psychosomatic symptoms and ailments. When the possibility of a psychosomatic illness diagnosis is gently proposed to the patient, it is often met with rage: *How dare you insinuate I am making this up or have an imaginary illness!* As long as I am reassured that the patient is getting the best medical treatment for the condition, I take the psychological route.

The Case of Myra

Myra and her husband came for treatment after being married for six years. They have a two-year-old infant. Their primary complaint is that they have not had sex since they had their baby. Myra explains that the reason they don't have sex is because she has a respiratory disease and has to be very careful about what she eats and where she sleeps in order to ensure that her house is germ free. She claims that any breach of sterility can result in a respiratory infection that can lead to suffocation. Myra demands that her husband sterilize the house, make sure all the dishes are cleansed properly, and that cooking pots do not in any way touch the dishes or other pots.

Myra's husband recently become very angry at her for trying to control the way he drives and for using his iPhone to make calls while she was explaining what needed to be done in the house. That night he had a dream that he heard a big bang. It was an airplane crash. Everyone was in shock; people were screaming and yelling. It was a gruesome situation, and everyone was horrified. During an individual session with the husband, it became clear that the dream represented the fear that if he ever expresses his needs to Myra, or confronts her in any way, let alone demands sex, it is tantamount to a big explosion. "She has me by the balls. I am terrified that my actions will cause her illness to flare up. Last time I said anything that upset her I had to rush her to the emergency room."

Myra, intuitively sensing the possibility that I was going to bring up the sexual issue and how this unmet need causes frustration for her husband, preempted me by calling the morning of their next appointment, saying that she could not make the session because she had not been able to sleep all night and was in excruciating pain. I interpreted to her husband that she is enacting the same scenario with me and with him, that my demands also drive her to illness and that she coerces both of us to go along with her for fear that we will endanger her and make her sick.

In a conjoint session, I made it clear that I would not bring up any issues that were disturbing to Myra until she felt she was ready. I also reminded her that the reason for treatment was to work on the marriage. At this point, she started to cough and said she was having troubling swallowing. I reminded her of her suffocating mother, who used to throw food down Myra's throat, forcing her to eat, and tell her negative things about herself. Myra complained that "I feel like someone has a vice grip on my torso, and I can't breathe too well, even after being on all my medications. I feel like an old lady who used to smoke, someone with emphysema who has no oxygen."

I reassure Myra that I am not abusive, that I care about her and her marriage, that I am trying to open up her airways, not block them. I take every opportunity to interpret the unconscious material, to help make the unconscious conscious. When Myra sensed I was going to make demands of her, she would either cancel or say she was too ill. The big bang came when her husband reported he had to go on a business trip. This resulted in her screaming, yelling, and indulging in out-of-control behavior, "How can you leave me? Can't you see I'm sick? Who will take care of me?" When he brought up the prospect of a caretaker, she became completely hysterical. What was he thinking, bringing in all these germs from the outside?

It was imperative that as therapist I match the words with Myra's experience. For instance, when she started to choke after a demand was made of her, I reminded her of how suffocating her mother was, to the point where Myra couldn't breathe. When she referred to fear of contamination, I placed it within the context of having sex with her husband. I mentioned how this could relate to fear of being contaminated not only by her husband's penis, but by my interpretations.

Discussion

Psychosomatic illness is expressed through various physical, biological, and mental influences—which often include physical symptoms that are mainly, but not exclusively, operative with histrionic individuals. Among these physical symptoms are chronic anxiety, depression, social phobias, fear of strangers, and obsessive-compulsive habits. The main dynamic is splitting and projective identification. The phobic histrionic masterfully coerces her object into complete submission and obedience to her. Myra is an interesting composite of a histrionic in that her diagnosis would fit within the realm of obsessive-compulsive disorder proper, given that she is obsessed with dirt, germs, and contamination. However, unlike the obsessive-compulsive, the more dominant features are her parasitic dependency and neediness. Given this history, I believe it is fair to refer to her as a disappearing woman, one who has disappeared not only from her role as mother, wife, and patient, but also from herself. Fortunately, Myra loved the analytic process, read widely, and eventually learned not to fear that my interpretations would suffocate her.

THE UNAVAILABLE WOMAN

The unavailable woman is a first cousin of the disappearing woman. I include them in the cluster of narcissistic and obsessive-compulsive types because of their icy coldness, aloofness, and matter-of-fact attitude. The unavailable women is the user, the abuser. She is callous, domineering, and judgmental, lacks empathy, and has little or no regard for the feelings of others. She is totally self-absorbed and sees men as part objects, there to service her needs. She often chooses borderline men—men who do not have a sense of self and are continually trying to prove they exist through their enactments with the unavailable women. *She would shop and shop until she depleted all our funds and drove us to bankruptcy. I begged her to be more prudent. The more desperate I got, the more deprived she felt and the more she shopped. I finally had to divorce her.*

The Case of Jackie

Jackie, an executive administrator, entered into treatment because of issues she was having with her co-workers. They complained that she never listened to their complaints, that she did not respond to their messages or emails, and would keep people waiting on hold forever. Jackie recognized that these complaints involved issues similar to those with men. She had mastered the skill of keeping men on hold and teasing them with her sexuality. She used them for her own self-serving purposes, but then pulled away at any sign of intimacy. When they got fed up or had enough, they would dump her.

The central feature of this case is that Jackie felt no shame, guilt, or remorse. If a man kept calling and leaving messages, Jackie would not respond until she felt like it. "They deserved what they got. I needed to be the center of his universe, and I was insanely jealous at the sight or even a mention of another woman. Now I don't give a crap. I have had them, done them, been there, been through the hurt, the rejection, the betrayal, and don't want it anymore. It leads to nothing but pain and heartbreak. I used to overreact and become overly dependent, emotional, sexually seductive, and clingy. I was in need of constant reassurance and extremely dependent. Now I am totally removed and use men in the way they used me! I met this man on the Internet, a nice man, extraordinarily well to do. He seems crazy about me. I have him take me to dinner, buy me gifts, get tickets to concerts, and when it comes to making love, I just do it to keep him to use him."

When asked why she responds the same way to her co-workers since she does not have the same vengeful attitude toward them, her response was, "It is because I like to be in control. I like to be needed. I like for people to come after me!" This kind of response opens up an entire array of opportunities for the therapist to explore the difficulty that a narcissist like Jackie has in allowing herself to be dependent on others. That they "need" her feeds and fuels her omnipotence and grandiose self.

The Case of Richard and the Unavailable Woman

Richard, a very successful trial attorney, came into session feeling a great deal of shame and embarrassment for being in a three-year relationship with a woman who is unavailable.

I invited Kathy to dinner at a very posh, upscale restaurant and was delighted when she accepted right away, without giving me all the excuses or saying "Let me think about it" or "Let me check out my schedule." She just said, "Yes, okay." When I arrived at the restaurant, my mouth dropped open. There she was, with two of her girlfriends. She said she hoped I didn't mind. One friend had just come in from out of town and only had a few days, and the other called and wanted to join us. As usual, I was polite and went along. But when the bill came, I noticed no one moved or even made a gesture. So, of course, I ended up paying for all four of us. I was pissed as hell.

When we finally got our reservations to go to Hawaii, again I was thrilled because this time I knew we would spend time together, talk, have fun, and just do stuff. The first night after checking into the hotel, we were at the pool, and I kept noticing her running back to her cell phone. I asked who she was talking to and she said it was her mother; her mother wasn't feeling well and she had to check up on her. Well much to my dismay, it was not her mother. It was one of her old boyfriends! How did I know? When she was in the shower, I checked her messages and found a text and several calls back and forth. I was livid. When she got out of the shower, I confronted her about her lies and she started to laugh, "Oh," she said, "the problem with you, Richard, is that you are just too jealous!" I know she's right. I do get very jealous, and I know that is a big problem I have. I also know I should dump her, but I can't. She is like an albatross around my neck and the same things keep happening again and again.

Discussion

Richard presents many unresolved oedipal issues, mainly maternal fusion with a mother from whom he has never achieved separation-individuation. His masochistic tendencies, which make him embrace unavailable women, are a reflection of bonding with familiar, painful objects. The interplay between Richard and the unavailable woman is very similar to what Fairbairn describes: how one forever remains faithfully and loyally attached to a bad internal object. Richard is an example of a man who gets wrapped up in the distorted and delusional world of narcissistic, unavailable women, and is predisposed to identify with their negative projections.

When Kathy "disappears," or mistreats or abuses Richard, he feels like a nothing. Instead of dumping Kathy after she pulls all these stunts, as most men would, he stays around for more because she keeps him entrapped. Many of Richard's friends ridicule him and cannot understand why an intelligent, competent man would stay with a woman they would not wish on their worst enemies. Fusion with the maternal object is a most powerful force in Richard's object world and compels him repeatedly to choose women like his mother—women who make promises and keep him in a state of object wanting but never object attaining.

Perhaps even more most important is how Kathy, the unavailable woman, has brilliantly mastered the art of projection. She knows precisely how to hook into Richard's area of vulnerability, or V-spot, with skill and precision. Thus, when she accused him of being jealous, she was off the hook. In *The Narcissistic/Borderline Couple* and other publications, I describe how one person (e.g., a narcissist) can project a negative feeling into another (e.g., a borderline), who then identifies or over-identifies with that which is being projected, also known as the process of dual projective identification (Lachkar 2004b, 2008a, 2008b, 20011). In Richard's case, the therapist may respond: "She accused you of being jealous, so you started to retreat and succumb to her projection that it was bad to be jealous? What is wrong with being jealous? Yes, you were jealous, as would anyone be in that situation!"

THE OBSESSIVE-COMPULSIVE DISAPPEARING WOMAN

Obsessive-compulsive women operate at multiple levels of splitting from their objects. Instead of forming attachments with lovers, boyfriends, and friends, they replace this with time, money, objects, and compulsive work as priorities. This includes a very punitive and severe superego that not only demands perfection in others but within oneself. Obsessive-compulsive women are extremely critical of others and notice every trace of imperfection. In a number of cases, the woman will make the man feel like an outsider, as if he doesn't count and is not a number one priority in her life.

In her role as lover, the obsessive-compulsive woman disappears into libidinally detached replacement objects. These women give precise attention to detail, are mechanical and, although successful in their careers, stifle all emotionality and creativity. These women remain forever loyal to their compulsive martyrdom. They complain of their workaholism, their anal-retentive qualities, how difficult it is to give, to share, to be intimate—and that they virtually have no time for these activities. *It's been six months since we've had sex.* Others exhibit the typical obsessive-compulsive disorder patterns discussed in chapter 6—a preoccupation with order and cleanliness and a horror of dirt and contamination, to the exclusion of their love objects. Still others may turn to an obsession with illness as a means to withdraw or "disappear" from their intimate relationships.

THE CROSS-CULTURAL DISAPPEARING WOMAN

As we did with the disappearing male, we look to another culture—mainly to Japanese society in this case—to get a perspective on the cross-cultural disappearing female. Today many Japanese women are refusing to marry. They do not want to be put into a position of subservience to their husbands. Modern-day Japanese women are turning more and more away from the traditional image of home and children and choosing to live alone as an alternative life style. Although many traditional Japanese women still stay home to take care of the finances, the home, their children, and their husbands, Japanese women have moved away from home and hearth to a cathexis of material objects. I recount my own memories of visiting Japan, observing driven women frantically running to department stores in droves, as if they were going to meet with their long-lost lovers. Kernberg (1995) would consider this a perversion, where materialism and devotion to objects become the replacement for love. Even though Japanese men are increasingly looking to women for leadership and guidance, there is still much resistance to this trend. In the corporate world, it is unusual to find a high-ranking female official or corporate executive.

Before Japan's economic boom, Japanese woman were mainly married housewives who had total control over the household, the children, the finances, and had no need or plans to work outside the home. Contemporary Japanese women are going through a massive social, cultural, and economic shift, leaving a residue of teenage girls obsessed with shopping, material objects, and sexual promiscuity. A recent concern in Japan is the rise of a secular pop culture force encouraging risky behavior among teens—that of engaging in *enjo kōsai*—sex with elderly men. According to Veronica Chambers, author of *Kickboxing Geishas* (2007), these men offer gifts ranging from money and expensive items such as Rolex watches to Chanel and Louis Vuitton designer purses as a reward for sexual favors. Some of these girls are seen wearing short shirts without underwear, and going without showering to make their tans last longer, even though they "were rumored to smell" (p. 10). This defies all conventions and traditions because Japan is a shame culture, is group oriented rather than individualistic, and traditionally relies on hierarchical social relationships. For generations, Japan has been a culture that adheres to conformity; anyone who does not conform is shamed and an considered an outsider by the group—*tatemae-honne* (appearance, concern for what others think, saving face).

Chambers confirms that even though Japanese pop culture has been in existence for decades, Japanese women are turning their rebellion into a full-blown revolution that is impacting the entire culture—an outburst that is tied to identification with American idols. Chambers asks why Japanese girls are "shaming" their parents by wearing 10-inch heels, short mini shirts, sporting huge red lips, and even sewing their lips to resemble Japan's iconic Hello Kitty symbol. Traditionalists are shocked and horrified by the rise of "Citi Girls," who are not a far cry from prostitutes.

Why this sudden break from tradition, whereby the Japanese woman no longer accepts the traditional female role and refuses to take a subservient position to men? *You want shame? Here it is in your face* (a collective group fantasy of projective identification). I interpret these extreme behaviors as manic defenses. Girls who envy Hollywood stars not only mimic them but "become them" through caricatures. Have these girls become the symbolic brandishing swords of revolution, the new implants of a society of plastic women acting in robotic concert in an attempt to escape their pacifistic, repressed society?

From a psychohistorical perspective, one might interpret that these young girls have moved away from the image of the peaceful, harmonious chrysanthemum to that of the vagina/sword—no longer objects to compel men but to repel them. They have relinquished old roles and have spurred the emerging trend of women no longer wanting to stay home and raise children. In fact, the prime minister of Japan was brutally criticized when he referred to Japanese women as "birth machines." Maybe their message is a wake-up call for Japanese fathers and husbands to "come home" from their workplaces and learn how to relate to the newly independent Japanese woman before she "disappears" entirely.

SUMMARY

This chapter has shifted focus from the disappearing male to the disappearing female. It strives to legitimize and provide justification for men who have been abused, violated, and have experienced the same kinds of aggression and violations from women that women have long experienced and continue to experience. Being dumped goes both ways. Men who deal with disappearing women suffer gravely from being dismissed, betrayed, and mistreated physically, emotionally, and psychologically. This is not to disregard genuine reasons that women have to dump a man who is physically or emotionally abusive to them—such as destructive borderline men, sociopaths, pathological liars, or malignant narcissists. The cases described in this chapter are about men who have a desperate need for a close intimate relationship, and have basic, healthy needs that are not violent or destructive. But these needs are deliberately ignored by the unfeeling female partners they choose.

While the physically and emotionally disappearing women described in this chapter may not have clear and concise full-blown personality disorders, most exhibit some of the fundamental characteristics of these disorders. They show symptoms and mechanisms of defense, including withdrawal, isolation, abandonment, anxiety, splitting, and projective identification. Furthermore, they all share aspects of aggression, cruelty, lack of empathy, sadism, and envy—the very things that invade and infect the capacity to maintain love and intimacy.

The section on cross-culture describes "the dynamic of disappearance"—by illustrating a trend that is escalating in Japan as younger generations of woman "disappear" from their traditional roles and defy all the old rules.

Chapter Eleven

Treatment Techniques and Approaches

The treatment techniques presented in this chapter are consistent with the theoretical material detailed in this book and in many of my previous books and publications. I have modified the various approaches to treatment to meet the needs of the women who have been affected and traumatized by the disappearing male. Again, I must acknowledge profound gratitude to Melanie Klein, Otto Kernberg, Heinz Kohut, and many others mentioned previous. Without them I would not have the tools to help these women deal with their feelings of loss, mourning, and abandonment. Nor would I have the knowledge to diagnostically note the variances between a sudden physical withdrawal/disappearance and an intrapsychic withdrawal, which happens with the robotic or schizoid man.

The lists that follow include some of the more fundamental therapeutic functions.

ESSENTIAL THERAPEUTIC TOOLS

- Empathy
- Listening
- Containment
- Introspection
- Mirroring
- Bonding as self-object
- Transitional object to the transitional space
- Holding/containing/environmental mommy
- Sense of humor

BASIC TREATMENT SUGGESTIONS

- Bond with the woman; be warm, empathic, and mirror her experience.
- Listen, maintain good eye contact, and establish your authority by creating boundaries (goal of treatment, payment, cancellation policy, missed appointments).
- Avoid "too many words" and asking too many questions. The history will gradually unfold. Don't waste time; start right in on therapy.
- If you don't know what to say, remain silent or mirror back the experience of your patient.
- Even when you're silent, use body language and nonverbal communication to show you understand and are listening to what the patient is saying.
- Speak with meaning and conviction. Do not speak until you have something meaningful to say (clarification, interpretation, etc.).
- Interrupt the patient when she begins to ramble and remind her of the focus.
- Listen to the words, "the theme," as a pathway to discovery of the patient's internal objects.
- Never forget the value of humor, which can relieve tension and bring home a point to the patient.
- Set goals, reevaluate, and continually remind the patient of these goals.
- Be careful not to blame the patient, even though she identifies with a "bad internal object." Chances are she has played a part in the man's departure or withdrawal, but under no circumstances does she or any woman deserve this kind of mistreatment.
- Show empathy for the woman who has been dumped, and when the time is right introduce her to her internal objects (the rejecting/betraying object).
- Allow the patient time and space to express her pain.
- Be careful that the patient does not feel responsibility for the man's sudden departure and does not confuse depression with mourning and loss.
- Gradually show the patient that she ignored the red flags to ensure more awareness in the future.
- Stress the importance of functioning over being happy.
- Show the patient that even if she finds herself in the same predicament time after time, it still does not justify a man suddenly dumping her.
- Show the patient how awareness is different than self-blame.
- Show empathy, but be careful not to collude with the patient's shame or self-blame.
- Instead of using the word *depression*, refer to loss and mourning.
- Refer to the patient's fears, resistance, and anxiety.
- Summarize what has been accomplished at the end of each session, reevaluating treatment goals and salient issues.

Showing empathy, listening, understanding, and offering containment are all very important aspects of the therapeutic process, as is the therapist becoming a mirroring/self-object. I remember one supervisee in my group who felt guilty because she was collecting money from her patient while "all she was doing was listening." The group responded, "That is a therapeutic function!"

Often in treatment we feel stuck, not knowing what to say, how to respond. The women we treat may be flooded with emotion—anger, rage, sadness—to the extent that even the most experienced therapist has trouble containing the emotional pain. Sometimes our countertransference gets in the way, and we want to blurt out, "What! You are an intelligent, high-functioning woman. You of all people should have known better! Didn't you see he was a dreamer? Didn't you see he was your doctor and was violating ethical boundaries by dating you?" Of course, no therapist in her/his right mind would actually respond this way; instead we have analytic tools to guide us through this process. When in doubt, remain silent; the thought will come to you. When in doubt, mirror and reflect. When in doubt . . .

. . . LISTEN TO THE WORDS

Listening to the words is linked to the language of empathology. The words a patient chooses to use are often not random; they are an expression of the unconscious and must be listened to carefully. For example, each time a husband would see a photo of his wife's ex-husband, mayhem would follow. His V-spot would blow, and off he went. At the same time, he mentioned that he fixed thermostats. What a wonderful entrée to an interpretation! *I think you are telling us that each time your V-spot gets ignited, you blow, and there is no you to adjust the thermostat to handle your boiling inner feelings of jealousy.* A patient's use of words such as "robber, abuser, judge, betrayer" are indicators of the patient's state of mind. These words may have unconscious significance and help you open a pathway to her internal objects. *Yes, there can be a robber, but there can also be an internal part of yourself that robs you. Yes, there can be an external man who is very critical and judgmental, but there can also be a judgmental part of you that self-persecutes. Yes, there can be an external man who betrays you, makes you promises, and never comes through; but there can also be an internal betrayer, part of you that holds back and finds excuses for not moving forward.*

I am reminded of a female bookkeeper who was tired of her job and felt it was monotonous and boring. We discussed the possibility of her making a career change, but for several months she resisted searching for new possibilities that would bring her more success and gratification. Meanwhile, she and her friends would gather together and do crystal readings. "I just love the crystals: they are so clear and so beautiful," she told me. To this I responded,

"Yes, you can look at the crystals and admire them, or you could become a crystal." Her response: "But if I did become the crystal then I would be the subject of everyone's envy, and this would mean I would get attention. And you know how ashamed I feel when I get attention."

I cannot emphasize enough the importance that humor plays in psychotherapy. Just don't overdo it. Humor can be highly therapeutic and healing. In spite of the trauma and pain these woman experience after being abruptly left for reasons they often cannot fathom, it is essential that you appeal to their sense of humor as you proceed through therapy. Humor is often relieving and spurs healing. It disperses tension and opens up a new emotional space. Humor takes the edge off the trauma and transforms anxiety, putting it into the realm of the absurd and ridiculous rather than the bad and persecutory.

One woman was so distraught over the abrupt breakup of a relationship that at the end of the session she said she did not want to leave and asked if she could spend the night here. Instead of saying how out of the question and how unethical it would be, I replied, "Of course, here we provide the finest service. But did you make a reservation? Because right now we're at 100 percent occupancy?" A man upset about paying for his therapy says that I am no more than a prostitute. I tell him, "Actually a prostitute makes more money than I do!" Never forget your sense of humor!

TREATMENT PSYCHODYNAMICS

With the disappearing male syndrome, we see how certain dynamic mechanisms (grandiosity, entitlement, guilt, withdrawal) can arouse states of unworthiness and nonexistence in the women who have been abandoned (shame, blame, envy, abandonment, and persecutory anxieties). To address these dynamics, I find Melanie Klein offers us the most valuable methods and insights into understanding the distortions, delusions, and miscommunications involved. Drawing mainly on such concepts as splitting, projection, and projective identification, she moves into two major positions, the paranoid position and the schizoid position. Below are a few examples, which then take us into the three phases of treatment. The psychodynamics that follow are an integral part of our therapeutic tools.

Splitting

Patient: *I just want to divorce my wife, get rid of her. I am so bored and no longer feel the excitement I used to have!*

Therapist: *This is not about divorcing your wife; this is about divorcing a part of yourself that you cannot tolerate.*

Projective Identification

Patient: *I tried to hug him but he pushed me away. I felt so crushed and rejected. I started to sob nonstop.*

Therapist: *But if you take his pushing you away personally, you are not available to see that he is confusing suffocation with love. Your tears would suffocate him even more.*

P: *Then he would say, "Oh, don't give me that psychobabble stuff you learned from your therapist."*

Th: *If he says that, you can say, "Honey, I knew this when I was twelve years old. Don't you think I knew the difference between little boys who shied away from little girls who tried to get close and the boys who didn't?"*

The Bad Breast/Good Breast

The world is a terrible place vs. the world is a wonderful place. "There are no worthwhile men in the world" (bad breast), as opposed to "there are plenty of fish in the sea" (good breast).

Patient: *Nothing I do is good enough. I cook, I take care of the kids, I entertain his family, his friends. I'm sexy! I'm passionate. I feel so devalued and unappreciated!*

Therapist: *So no matter how much you try to please him, he coerces you into being the bad-breast mommy.*

Paranoid-Schizoid Position

Patient: *Everything that has gone wrong is because of her. She reminds me of my mother. She never gives me credit for anything, and I blame her for everything that goes wrong. She gets me so upset I don't know what to do. Should I stay married or should I divorce her?*

Therapist: *While you are in this state of blaming/attacking, it's not a good idea to make any major decisions* (primitive defenses get in the way of seeing the "real relationship").

The Depressive Position

Patient: *I feel so sad all the time. I go around crying, depressed.*

Therapist: *No, you are not depressed; you are dealing with normal states of sadness and taking more responsibility for your actions. This is a good time, where growth and progress occur and where reparation can be made.*

Even with all the tools and techniques available, the most skilled therapist can find it challenging to confront the spurned woman, and give her insight into her participation in the abandonment without making her feel she is to blame or at fault for the man's disappearance. To confront the women too soon can precipitate a rapprochement crisis. Even the less seasoned therapist knows to hold back observations while giving the woman with a bleeding heart the space and time to express her hurt and pain. The woman has been traumatized and deprived and is desperate. Men who mistreat women by disappearing in an unwarranted, unfeeling way have violated the women's "love rights."

He kept calling and calling after we met for coffee. He said I was the woman he had been waiting for his entire life. I was so thrilled that after being alone for so long, here was a man who desired me. He told me again and again how beautiful, sexy, and smart I was and that he had finally found a woman with beauty and brains. But he never asked me out. I realize now that he was the unavailable man, and I should have cut him off as soon as I saw the telltale signs. Instead I kept waiting for him to make a move.

A love relationship is one of the most intimate, sacred bonds imaginable and the closest to the mother/child relationship. There are some behaviors that are simply not acceptable. In addition, there are also some women who are blindsided and go into total ego dysfunctionality, where primitive defenses are operative (idealization, grandiose thinking, delusions, magical thinking, omnipotent denial). For these reasons I have developed three phases of treatment as a means of integrating the therapeutic process.

THE THREE PHASES OF TREATMENT

Phase One: Chaos, Confusion, and Splitting

This phase parallels Klein's paranoid-schizoid position, which represents a fragmented, chaotic state of mind in which one is not receptive to confrontation, interpretation, or responsibility for one's actions. This phase is rife with splitting, blaming, attacking, shaming defenses, uncontrollable rage, and desire for revenge. In some situations, aggression and rage can be turned inward: *It is all my fault.* During this phase the patient feels paralyzed, immobilized, unhappy, and unable to function. The therapist as the container then responds, "The focus should not be on happiness but more on functioning. Even though you don't feel like driving or going to work or the gym, you can still function." This phase highlights the containing aspect of the therapist, who at the same time must show compassion for the patient's state of mind.

Both these ends of the spectrum are operative in phase one. This position represents the earliest state of mind where primitive defense dominates: guilt, shame, deprivation, victimization, control, oedipal issues all come to the fore. The therapeutic challenge is to avoid making the woman feel that she is responsible for the abuse, mistreatment, or sudden abandonment, while simultaneously opening the pathway to letting her know how she may have missed the danger signs. It is a space that acts as a safe containing environment in which the therapist provides such helpful functions as mirroring and empathic attunement.

One woman was absolutely devastated when her husband of ten years suddenly served her with divorce papers. "I was so stunned, I couldn't think, couldn't move, and felt totally paralyzed. I did not know what to tell the kids why daddy suddenly left." During this stage the therapist was quite aware of and very sensitive to the patient's feelings and did not confront the patient about her participation. She had been retreating from sex within the marital relationship and had not noticed her husband's increasing withdrawal and distance. Her unawareness was a major factor in prompting her husband's sudden abandonment. At this stage, it would have been much too soon to confront the patient's participation, which requires containment on the part of the therapist. Even when the patient reveals a traumatic history, it must be emphasized that the man had no right to suddenly or abruptly abandon her and the family.

Phase Two: A Transitional Phase

This phase marks the beginning of bonding with the therapist as a reparation object, which will wean her away from her bad internal objects. It is a transitional state in which the therapist emerges as the a mirroring/self-object and acts as an environmental containing object. This allows the therapist to lead the patient away from living emotionally "inside" the object to living "outside" the object—a state of "not knowing." This phase marks the emergence of "twoness," moving away from fusion to a state of separation-individuation and immersion inside the mental state of the lost object. *Where is he? Where did he go? Does he think about me? Is he with someone else? What did I do wrong?* In this phase, the woman is more aware of how she needs to separate herself from the internal bad objects with which she has identified. During this phase, the therapist helps her to realize that awareness is not the equivalent of self-blame but more about learning from experience, teaching her how to pay attention to what she intuitively sensed and perceived at the onset of the relationship. *I knew he was a player, a womanizer, but I thought with me it would be different.*

It is the beginning of more in-depth analytic work, whereby the therapist introduces the patient's internal objects, her grandiose self, and her betraying/abandoning self. *Yes, there can be a husband or lover who suddenly abandons you, but there can also be an internal part of yourself that abandons you. You did not trust your perceptions; nor were you aware of how your husband was withdrawing from you, distancing himself, spending more and more time at work. And you withdrew sex from him.*

Phase Three: The Depressive Position

The depressive position is a state of mourning wherein the patient is able to take responsibility for her own actions. There is less splitting, more self-awareness, and a growing ability to learn from experience. It is a time for reparation and for the patient to embrace her guilt, accept it, and deal with loss and sadness. Moving into the more whole and integrated depressive position allows the patient to begin to take responsibility for her own wrongdoings. There is a diminishment of envy, shame, blame, attacking, revenge, magical thinking, and the desire to make reparation for the damage that has been done.

It is very important that in this phase the state of mourning is not confused with depression; rather, it is a healthy state of mind that marks the ability to deal with sadness and loss.

> Patient: *I have been seeing you now for three months and I feel even worse. I am very depressed!*
>
> Therapist: *No, you are not depressed. What you are feeling is normal, and you must continue to function. I know you feel paralyzed and immobilized but you can still keep moving, as you do in your aerobics class. You may not feel happy, but at least you will know you are functioning.*

It is in this final stage that the therapist can introduce the patient to her internal bad object and point out her tendency to identify with the bad object—e.g., the unavailable object, the rejecting object, the betraying object. Often, the abandoned woman has bonded with the wronged self, a blaming/attacking/persecutory self, a betrayed self, a deprived self, an insatiable self, a robbed self. *I always blame myself when a man suddenly disappears from my life. My first impulse is to ask myself what I did wrong.*

In treating women who have been left high and dry by the disappearing male, the therapist's job is to help her link her bad internal and external objects. This has enormous merit in the treatment of women who have been dumped. It helps the woman get her control back. *No, we can't control all the betrayers, the abusers, the deceivers out there. But we can control the internal betrayer, abuser, deceiver—the part of you that betrays yourself, that does not trust or listen to your perceptions then gets seduced by the disappearing, unavailable man. When you work out at the gym, you need to find your core. It's the same with your mind. You must strengthen your mental core.*

Eventually in treatment the abandoned woman begins to question why she chooses the same types over and over again—men who are not available, men who torment her. These are the rejecting objects, the depriving objects, the unavailable objects, the withholding objects, the abusive/tormenting or sadistic objects, the idealized objects, etc. *He is just like my father, always making promises but never following through.* What follows is an example of how these dynamics are applied in clinical practice.

The Case of Lisa

Patient: *I just don't get it! What's wrong with me? I am a college graduate, have a great job, and yet I can't find a man who wants to be with me. They all leave.*

Therapist: *But each time you thought they would be different and stay.*

P: *Yes, of course. They all came across as very charming and very much interested in having a long-term, loving relationship with me.*

Th: *What about the married man you dated for two years?*

P: *That was a disaster He kept promising me he was going to get a divorce, that he couldn't stand his wife, that I was the woman he wanted to live with and spend the rest of his life with.*

Th: *How did you feel when so much time went by and he didn't even contact a divorce attorney?*

P: *Feel! How did you expect me to feel? I felt stupid, like I'm an idiot for putting up with this crap and his unfulfilled promises. He was just using me! And I was blindsided.*

Th: *But you did see it. There were some very early signs.*

P: *Yes, you are right, I did see some signs. Like the first Valentine's Day he did not even send me a card and spent a weekend away with his wife.*

Th: *That must have been very painful.*

P: *Painful!!! But I rationalized it, thinking he just wanted to placate her before dropping the bomb. I always made excuses for him.*

Th: *First of all, Lisa, you are not stupid; nor are you an idiot. You've fallen into a trap that many women fall into. Second, you were bonded to him and were feeling so lonely and desperate you wanted to believe his lies were the truth. Third, no matter what you did or how you got hooked, what he did was wrong. Outright wrong. He had no right to keep you on hold, lying to you, making promises he could not keep.*

P: *I still feel like a big fool.*

Th: *No! In no way are you a fool. But I might add that you do have a history of falling in love with the unavailable man, men who dangle a carrot in front of you and offer you promises but are unreachable. But the real unavailable object is* you*! You gave up a part of yourself—the need to be loved, to be cherished, to be valued for who you are and not a little girl waiting for a daddy to come home.*

P: *You're right. My last boyfriend wasn't married, but he kept promising me commitment and never followed through. The one before was an alcoholic and was more committed to his gin than to me.*

Th: (silent as she goes through a barrage of past relationships)

P: *I know what you're waiting for. Yes, it has to do with my father doesn't it? My dad always promised he would take me out for my birthday, take me places like shopping or to Disneyland. But he always had excuses, and other things always seemed to be of more importance.*

Th: *Yes, you nailed it! This is not your fault, and you should not take the blame for the past. Rather, learn from the experience that you do have a proclivity to attach yourself to men like your father, those who promise but cannot fulfill.*

P: *I confess that other types of men bore me.*

Th: *They bore you because they don't offer you the challenge of working through these dynamics.*

P: *Yes, you're right. But at least I feel I am alive and the dream somehow keeps me going.*

Th: *It is not the dream that keeps you going. It is the pain and the memories of abandonment and deprivation (being bonded to the pain). As bad as the pain is, it is still better than the emptiness and loneliness that you would momentarily feel if you had left the relationship sooner.*

P: *Hmmm . . . bonded to the pain. So my fantasy is that if I repeat the same thing again and again maybe something will change.*

Th: *Right on! Yet, it doesn't change. The only change that can occur is right here because I am here for you. I hope you will find our work challenging and that you won't find me boring.*

P: *No! Of course not! Actually, I never really thought about my attachment to these men in this way. So I guess I'm not stupid then, am I?*

Th: *Certainly not! You have provided some amazing insights.*

P: *Great!*

Th: *See you next week.*

P: *Bye!*

Discussion

The therapist was cautious not to introduce Lisa to her own unavailable object too soon. She uses the language of empathology to gradually confirm Lisa's experience and to move Lisa away from the idea that she is stupid or dumb. As treatment progresses, the therapist gradually introduces her to the "Mother of Pain." As bad as the unavailable man is and the pain Lisa feels at his abandoning her, at least she feels a sense of aliveness and does not have to face her aloneness. Of her own accord, Lisa's associations lead to an unavailable father who had similarly made promises but never kept them. The therapist brings Lisa to the awareness that the repetition of moving from one unavailable man to another is not going to resolve her conflicts (repetitive compulsion). Instead the therapist introduces herself as a new self object, someone who is available and will offer Lisa the challenges she is desperately seeking.

SUMMARY

This chapter on treatment techniques and approaches draws mainly on object relations and self psychology, theories that encourage movement. Object relations provide us with the ebb and flow between the inner and outer self, between the bad external object world and identification with a bad inner object world that not only shapes the choices people make but helps explain why they stay bonded to painful, conflictual relationships.

As a dancer, I love movement and technique and the blending of the two. In therapy I love the movements that flow back and forth between the inner and outer selves; between partners via dual projective identification; between the dynamics of guilt and shame, envy and jealousy; between domination and submission, reality and magical thinking. I love the empathic stance that Kohut provides, and admire the confrontational aspects of Klein that move from the intersubjective world to the world of delusions and distortions and knowing these oppositional approaches can do the dance together. I love the freedom of the therapist to move from being empathic, sympathetic, and understanding to suddenly confronting the patient with laser-like precision while simultaneously relieving the patient of self-blame and persecutory anxiety. I also love allowing space for awareness as learning from experience overcomes self-blame and shame. I love how the three phases of treatment move back and forth interchangeably while at the same time moving into a higher stage of development. Mostly, I love the experience of observing the patient move away from states of the unmentalized experience to self-awareness and to opening up a new window of opportunity. *I am no longer a dumped woman!*

Chapter Twelve

Epilogue

Brave New Worlds

PARTNERING ON THE INTERNET

We cannot discuss the disappearing male—or disappearing female—syndrome without acknowledging the formidable new way people are hooking up within the dating world. The Internet is tailor made for career-oriented types and single parents who don't have time to spend finding a partner through the usual channels. It's also a boon for the shy, lonely, and older crowds who eschew the bar or club scene. The Internet can be a very practical and efficient way of meeting people. It is important to recognize that Internet dating is no longer the elephant in the room. It's accepted and is here to stay.

People from all over the world are meeting, dating, and communicating online via dating sites, Facebook, Twitter, chat rooms, blogs, IMs, etc. It is no wonder therapists are seeing more cross-cultural couples as people from all over the world chat, mix and match, and carry on virtual romances that eventually continue in real venues. People are hooking up with partners from different cultures and ethnic groups, with little thought that they bring to these couplings their own nationalistic flags, their often disparate traditions regarding love and marriage, religion, the treatment of women, and child-rearing practices, to name a few. The dynamics of dating and getting to know another person take on an entirely different shape when not conducted face to face.

In the United States the relationship takes priority. We emphasize the importance of love as a primary force for marrying and having children. In other cultures different things take precedence: one's job, duty to country, duty to parents and elders, etc. There are not too many couple therapists or couple clinics sprouting up in Baghdad, Saudi Arabia, or even in modern-day Japan. Children grow and leave the nest but, ideally, couples are "forever." Based on many interviews with rabbis, priests, ministers in the United States, I believe almost all clergy are in accord that the wife/husband comes first and has priority over other relationships. I am reminded of the situation in which a Japanese businessman was supposed to celebrate his wife's birthday but cancelled at the last minute to go out with a business partner. The man who gives up his wife's birthday for his business partner blatantly prioritizes his work over his wife.

While there are many positive aspects of Internet dating, it does have a dark side. People can pretend to be anyone on the Internet. Sometimes the pretense is just the 20-year-old photo in one's profile on an online dating site. But there are horror stories of potential soul mates who turn out to be swindlers, cheaters, liars, and even predators. Therapists, whose analytical training has heightened their ability to decode messages, discover unconscious meanings, and decipher symbolic representations, should warn their patients of potential red flags by alerting them to hidden meanings in profiles and even in the profile names. Some profiles may on the surface appear quite affable, pleasant, or congenial; but underneath they may convey an entirely different message. Take for example, the statement "My daughter means everything in the world to me!" Well, is that daughter a little girl? Is she a rebellious teenager who would be jealous of anyone who could someday take her mother's place? Is she married? Does the daughter have a life of her own? Is her father so fused with his daughter that he may not be able to make room for a new love in his life? These are the kinds of things therapists can help men and women explore.

Female patients have told me tales of men who "insist" on picking them up at their homes on the first date, even after the woman mentions more than once that she would prefer to meet at a local public meeting place. It may sound precipitous on my part, but this type of persistence might very well signal trouble. I suggest to the woman that she pick up the danger sign that a man who can't take no for an answer may have a serious pathology. If he continues to persist, then she can say something like, "Nothing personal but I have my homeland security policy—never having a man come to my home the first time."

Unfortunately, indicators of potential danger are not clear and precise. There are no rules, merely guidelines. Let us take a moment to examine a few Internet dating profiles and how they could serve to give the dater indications about where the priorities of a person lie, even at first glance. This may sound a bit pejorative, which it is not meant to be; rather, it is designed to help guide the dater to become more aware.

Decoding Profile Examples

- The most important things are my kids—or Porsche, horse, dog, boat, working out (commitment phobic).
- On the first date I would like to hold hands and take a walk on the beach (poor boundaries).
- I don't know what to say about myself except my friends tell me I'm a nice guy (no sense of self).
- I am well shaven, just lost 54 pounds, moved in with my mother, and am looking to relocate (poor boundaries, low self-image).
- Looking for a woman who is independent and low maintenance (cheap).
- If your photo is more than twenty years old, I'm sure you were lovely then, but please don't bother to contact me (attacking).
- Mr. Nice Guy, been married four times, looking for my soul mate (idealist loser).
- I am looking for a place to relocate and lost my sunglasses last week (just plain loser).

Profile Names to Be Wary Of

- Noodle 2 (weak, passive, dependent)
- Run4URlife (scared)
- Sciddle Saddle (not serious)
- My Harley and Me (avoids intimacy)
- Born to Race (manic)
- Charmer (Don Juan type)
- Dreamer (delusional)
- Little boy names like Bobbie, Billie, Chuckie, Andy (Peter Pan types)

In contrast to the danger signs that can be embedded in some Internet names, there are more positive signals one may come across:

- Renaissance man (however, could also be a flaming narcissist)
- Likes to please (could also be a false self, obsequious and overly compliant)
- Looking for the love of my life
- Want someone to share my life with
- Have a zest for life and want someone to share its joys with me
- Adult male names like Robert, Charles, Andrew

COSMETIC SURGERY

This book would not be complete without mentioning cosmetic surgery—an option that has exploded in the last couple of decades. Woman are increasingly abandoning their "old" faces and their wrinkles and making themselves over, either partially and completely. While this is also happening among men who want to look younger so they can complete with people years their junior for jobs or look less severe (Botox can smooth away frown lines), women are more prone to seek cosmetic changes to make themselves more alluring or to feel better about themselves. The abandoned woman is most likely to be the recipient of cosmetic surgery to redeem herself after having her ego completely deflated by the disappearing male.

Today it's becoming almost normal in our clinical practices to treat women who are considering having cosmetic work done or who have already undergone a plethora of cosmetic procedures from Botox and other fillers to face lifts, breast implants, tummy tucks, eye lifts, etc. Cosmetic surgery has increased exponentially. Even 16-year-old and younger girls have opted to have their breasts augmented.

Cosmetic procedures no longer are kept secret. In fact, women seem to derive great pleasure from showing off their newly acclaimed treasures. *I'll show you mine if you show me yours.* Old bodies are constantly being rejuvenated in some way as people desperately strive to look younger and more vital. It is well known that many of these cosmetic surgeries are unnecessary. In some cases women become addicted to cosmetic interventions and end up looking like plasticized versions of themselves. In an effort to make themselves over, they go overboard and lose all perspective on who and what they are. Often the reasons for having these procedures are completely flawed. Because of this, I am including some diagnostic categories that might apply to women who seek cosmetic surgery to serve as guidelines and assessment measures for therapists and doctors alike.

The Narcissist

This personality type has great need for attention, fame, power, entitlement. In addition, the narcissist has grandiose, omnipotent expectations and strives for perfection. Aging is a gross narcissistic injury for many of these women for they have the unrealistic expectation that they should remain young and beautiful forever. They are difficult to treat because they have excessive entitlement fantasies and an idealized image of how things should be in the world, including how they should look.

The Borderline

These women feel ugly inside and turn to plastic surgery to obliterate their internal feelings of ugliness, shame, and deprivation. There is distortion and confusion between their inner and outer selves. *I feel dirty inside so I look ugly on the outside!* Borderlines have a great deal of pent-up rage and hostility and will act out their destructive behavior by projecting onto others. When betrayed or abandoned, they will resort to revenge, retaliation, and getting even with anyone whom they feel has wronged them. They often distort reality and believe their lies are the truth. Doctors beware! These are among the patients most likely to sue.

The Obsessive-Compulsive

They strive for perfection and are obsessed with cleanliness and orderliness. These are the control freaks who have a great deal of difficulty with dependency needs and trust. They can drive the doctor crazy with endless questions, which they repeat over and over again. Obsessive-compulsives are very anxious and will go to any extreme to make sure they understand every detail of the surgery before they proceed. They aim to be "dirt free," totally cleansed by perfect results.

The Depressed Personality

Nothing ever pleases or satisfies them or makes them happy. They are characterized by hatred turned inward. They tend to self-blame and attack when anything goes wrong. These are the victims, and thus are often not good candidates for surgery. Internal anger, which has turned into remorse and sadness, is felt to be ugly, and the depressed personality erroneously thinks that cosmetic surgery will be the solution. The depressed patient not only *feels* depressed, he *becomes* the depression.

The Histrionic

This is the forever-young patient, the one who can never be satisfied and can opt for one surgery after another. She is the little girl or the adolescent who has never grown up. Nor is she comfortable with her womanhood. She is seductive, flirtatious, and gets a false sense of self-esteem by attracting the attention of men.

The Passive-Aggressive

These are among the most difficult patients because they are the victims, the ones always delaying and putting things off. *I'll do it mañana.* Getting payment is difficult and tedious, and so is making appointment arrangements. *"How about next week?" "No, that won't work." "What about the week after?" "I think I might be able to squeeze that in. I'll let you know."* This is followed by numerous cancellations with endless excuses.

The Cross-Cultural Patient

The ethnic nose is the most common form of surgery for women who come to this country and want to have the westernized look. Doctors often overlook the fact that there is beauty in the distinct and unique quality of the nose. The Middle Eastern or Jewish nose is the most frequently remodeled. Eyelid surgery to remove the epicanthic fold that gives oriental eyes their beautifully distinctive look is also becoming more frequent.

The Malignant Narcissist

These patients are cautious and quite likely to sue. At the onset, they will tend to idealize the doctor as a savior, then later shift to revenge and anger because nothing done to them is ever good enough. They are often envious of the doctor and will distort and abuse the doctor's good intentions. The malignant narcissist feels entitled to get something back, perhaps because the results may not be as perfect as "God meant them to be."

The Malignant Borderline

These patients are also cautious and likely to sue. Malignant borderlines have antisocial features, no conscience, and will sue not so much out of entitlement but more out of revenge. They are most concerned with domination, control, and revenge. They are sometimes envious of the doctor and have the unconscious wish to destroy or sabotage even those who try to help them—mental health professionals, counselors, teachers, managers, lawyers, doctors, including, of course, cosmetic surgeons.

Although Otto Kernberg is not a plastic surgeon, he helps us understand how people with various disorders suffer from ego deficits, and that the first thing to go is the ego. The ego is the mechanism responsible for:

- Thinking (the victimized self can give one a distorted image of self and other)
- Reality testing (fantasy that surgery will be a cure all)
- Perception (idealization of the cosmetic surgeon as a miracle worker)
- Judgment (poor choices)

- The ability to tolerate anxiety (impulsiveness, the need for immediate gratification, difficulty dealing with disappointment if results are less than what is expected)

In debating the subject of plastic surgery with a colleague as being suitable for inclusion in this chapter, she stated, "It has applicability if the motivation behind the plastic surgery is clarified. In many cases it is the alienation of the true self to the false self." She also commented that, "Plastic surgery should enhance one's own beauty, not strive to make one younger" (Roberta Rinaldi, LCSW). Her frame of reference was Helen Mirren, a beautiful but "older" woman who does not try to look or act like a twenty-something-year-old.

In this brave new cosmeticized world of fillers, breast implantation, plumped lips, and born-again eyelids, women are mesmerized by pop culture and Hollywood stars. They pour into cosmetic surgeons' offices in droves, hoping that a new look and the disappearance of laugh lines, crow's feet, and sagging jowls will bring them the elusive happiness they seek. Many plastic surgeons confirm that "you can give them a new face and new breasts, but it does not resolve their underlying issues." Cosmetic surgeons are familiar with the narcissistic patient who may request many unnecessary surgeries. However, only recently have they started to pay greater attention to other diagnostic categories in assessing patients who seek cosmetic procedures.

In another form of "disappearance," many women's minds vanish to states of idealization that revere and idealize their beloved doctors who will save and rescue them from their sagging, aging world of wrinkles and age spots. They rely on Dr. Ponce de Leon to lead them to the fountain of youth and eternal satisfaction with who they are. This in no way is meant to undermine those with legitimate needs—e.g., those who require reconstructive surgery, those with a healthy desire to improve their looks, people whose work depends on how they look. The focus here is on those who become obsessed with and addicted to adjusting their looks or are seeking a process to change their lives in ways cosmetic surgery cannot possibly do. I recall one patient who wanted to look Britney Spears "and I don't care how many surgeries it will take." The Octomom is another woman who had "work" done in an attempt to look like Angelina Jolie. One renowned cosmetic surgeon I interviewed stated:

No one would ever have imagined when I became a surgeon, let alone a plastic surgeon interested making women more beautiful, that I would be linking my work to psychology. As time goes on and I have interviewed and performed surgery on vast numbers of women throughout the world, I begin to see how our medical field is inextricably linked to psychology. Having been in personal psychoanalysis for many years, I can see the benefits of making more accurate clinical and diagnostic assessments of potential pa-

tients because of the experience and knowledge I have gained from being on the couch.

CLOSING THOUGHTS

The plight of the abandoned woman, although a highly specialized area, is a very common theme and has been grossly overlooked in the literature. This book outlines various approaches and techniques useful in treating women who have loved, trusted, and ended up humiliated, shamed, betrayed, traumatized, and shocked by the sudden disappearance of a man. Many of these women are intelligent, highly educated, and high functioning and cannot believe they got duped and completely ignored the danger signs. This book also points out that the woman's traumatic or abusive past may contribute to her lack of awareness or "ego dysfunctionality," but that this still does not justify a man's violation of her "love rights."

Although this book is mainly for mental health professionals, much of the information and suggestions it contains have applicability for patients, parents, teachers, business professionals, physicians, and others who deal with disappearing male syndrome and those whom it affects. The chapter on cross-culture is also beneficial for politicians, government officials, historians, homeland security officials, and international scholars.

In the discussion of techniques, I have emphasized that psychotherapy is an art form which requires highly developed skills; yet it also requires the therapist's creativity and imagination. When a woman who has been victimized by the disappearing male leaves the therapy session, the hope is that she will feel embraced, contained, and have the newly gained insight that the world has not closed up on her but that a whole new window of opportunity has opened. Women must awaken to the reality that there are men who prey on women's vulnerability as caretakers and nurturers and must somehow find a way to band together to keep these admirable and endearing traits from turning them into victims.

Although we do not expect women in the dating world to carry a diagnostic manual with them or do a complete psychiatric mental status exam on every man they're with, we do hope to bring to their awareness the various personality types outlined in this book and alert women to the red flags and danger signs. *All he did on our first date was talk about himself.* Of course, we can offer only guidelines since life and diagnostic categories are not all black and white. But we can almost be sure that if a man acts like a narcissist on the first date, he will act that way on the second, and third.

Another aim of this book is to acknowledge and encourage the amazing perception of women. They are emotionally attuned to what is going on around them, and they must learn to trust their instincts and discernment.

Isn't it ironic that in a flash a women can recognize a handbag as a Louis Vuitton or Chanel knock-off, yet cannot recognize that the man they're with is a complete fake?

Women also must get over feeling the pressure to have sex. What most women don't recognize is that bonding emotionally is a precursor to having a satisfying sexual relationship—not the other way around. There are two reasons why women commonly capitulate: (1) because of feelings of desperation, frustration, loneliness, and deprivation for not having a man in her life, and (2) because of the fear that if she does not conform to the man's desire, he will leave or abandon her. The irony is that in most instances he will leave or abandon her anyway since she no longer presents a challenge. Outwardly, the man may respond with great excitement and enchantment; inwardly or unconsciously he may say to himself, "She is too needy, too desperate, can't contain, is not safe, can't be trusted."

I suggest that women learn to band together using the Internet as a forum. Women with similar problems should form support and therapy groups and use Internet chat rooms to connect with other women throughout the world to openly express and share their stories and feelings without shame—and with the knowledge they are not alone.

Finally, there are the societal issues. With changing customs and mores and the advent of the Internet, people no longer rely on face-to-face meeting places such as churches, synagogues, or social clubs to find a partner. Even friends or acquaintances no longer "fix up" people much, which used to be one of the most common and reliable ways to meet a trustworthy partner. One woman reportedly asked her friend of twenty years if she knew of any single men. The response was, "Why don't you go online? There are hundreds of single men." Hence, a disappearing society!

I have shared my clinical and professional experience in the hope that this book will help instill in women all over the globe the knowledge that they are entitled to the universal human right to be loved, cherished, and respected by men. For without us there would be no men!

Fini

Glossary

These terms are mentioned throughout this book and referenced in many of my previous publications.

Attunement: Attunement is the rhythm of the heart and soul as it blends with another person. According to Winnicott (1965), it is the mother/infant experience of togetherness, that special moment when the infant and mommy are one—in total harmony, bliss, and synchronicity. This beautiful moment of closeness takes place against the backdrop of dialectic tensions involving the dread of separateness. Whether it involves the mother and infant, the dancer and the pianist, the musician and the conductor, the painter and his canvas, or the patient and his analyst, there are two types of attunement: (1) the moment of togetherness and (2) sensing the rhythm and timing of the other.

Borderline Personality: This personality disorder designates a defect in the maternal attachment bond as an over-concern with the "other." Many have affixed the term "as-if personalities" to borderlines. This refers to their tendency to subjugate or compromise themselves. They question their sense of existence, suffer from acute abandonment and persecutory anxiety, and tend to merge with others in very painful ways in order to achieve a sense of bonding. Under close scrutiny and stress, they distort, misperceive, have poor impulse control, and turn suddenly against self and others (to attack, blame, find fault, and get even).

Containment: A term employed by Wilfred Bion, containment describes the interaction between the mother and the infant. Bion believed that all psychological barriers universally dissolve when the mind acts as receiver of communicative content, which the mother does in a state of reverie by using her own alpha function. Containment connotes the capacity to transform the data of emotional experience into meaningful feelings and thoughts. The mother's capacity to withstand the child's anger, frustrations, and intolerable feelings becomes the container for these effects. This can occur if the mother is able to sustain intolerable behaviors long enough to decode or detoxify painful feelings into a more digestible form.

Couple Transference: Couple transference is a term I devised to describe what happens during treatment when the partners jointly project onto the therapist some unconscious fantasy—e.g., making the therapist feel guilty for stopping the session on time, giving them a bill, not changing appointment times, etc. Together the partners form a folie à deux.

Cultural V-Spot: The cultural V-spot is a collectively shared archaic experience from the mythological or historical past that evokes painful thoughts and memories for the group, e.g., burning of the temple, loss of land to Israel, the expulsion of Ishmael to the desert with his abandoned mother, Hagar.

Depressive Position: This is a term devised by Melanie Klein to describe a state of mourning and sadness in which integration and reparation take place. In this state not everything is seen in terms of black and white. There is more tolerance, guilt, remorse, self-doubt, frustration, pain, and confusion. One is more responsible for one's action. There is the realization not of how things should be, but the way they are. As verbal expression increases, one may feel sadness but one may also feel a newly regained sense of aliveness.

Dual Projective Identification: Whereas projective identification is a one-way process, dual projective identification is a two-way process that lends itself to conjoint treatment. One partner projects a negative feeling onto the other, who then identifies or over identifies with the negativity being projected. *I'm not stupid! Don't call me stupid!*

Ego: The ego is part of an intrapsychic system responsible for functioning (thinking, reality testing, judgment). It is the mediator between the id and superego. The function of the ego is to observe the external world, preserving a true picture by eliminating old memory traces left by early impressions and perceptions.

Empathology: Empathology is a language I devised for talking to the eight different types of narcissists I delineated, using various communication styles applicable for each type. It is a term I abstracted from Heinz Kohut's concept of empathy. Empathology is an essential therapeutic technique in treating the narcissistic personality disorder.

Envy: Klein made a distinction between envy and jealousy. Envy is a part-object function and is not based on love. She considers envy to be the most primitive and fundamental emotion. It exhausts external objects, and is destructive in nature. Envy is possessive, controlling, and does not allow in outsiders.

Folie à deux: In general terms, folie à deux refers to Melanie Klein's notion of projective identification, whereby two people project their delusional fantasies back and forth and engage in a foolish "dance." The partners are wrapped up in a shared delusional fantasy, and each engages and believes in the outrageous scheme of the other. Usually the term applies to both oppositional and collusive couples. In some cases there is triangulation, which is a three-part relationship in which two people form a covert or overt bond against another member.

Guilt: Guilt is a higher form of development than shame. Guilt has an internal punishing voice that operates at the level of the superego (an internalized, punitive, harsh parental figure). There are two kinds of guilt: valid guilt and invalid guilt. Valid guilt occurs when the person should feel guilty. Invalid guilt comes from a punitive and persecutory superego.

Internal Objects: Internal objects result from an intrapsychic process whereby unconscious fantasies that are felt to be persecutory, threatening, or dangerous are denounced, split off, and projected. Internal objects emanate from the part of the ego that has been introjected. Klein believed that the infant internalizes good "objects" or the "good breast." However, if the infant perceives the world as bad and dangerous, the infant internalizes the "bad breast."

Jealousy: Jealousy, a higher form of development than envy, is a whole-object relationship whereby one desires the object but does not seek to destroy it or the oedipal rival (father and siblings—those who take mother away). Jealousy, unlike envy, is a triangular relationship based on love, wherein one desires to be part of or included in the group, family, clan, nation.

Manic Defenses: The experience of excitement (mania) offsets feelings of despair, loss, anxiety, and vulnerability. Manic defenses evolve as a defense against depressive anxiety, guilt, and loss. They are based on omnipotent denial of psychic reality and on object relations characterized by a massive degree of triumph, control, and hostility. Some manic defenses work in the ego.

Mirroring: This is a term devised by Heinz Kohut that describes the "gleam" in a mother's eye, which mirrors the child's exhibitionistic display. This maternal response to the child's narcissistic-exhibitionist displays confirms the child's self-esteem. Eventually these responses are channeled into more realistic aims.

Narcissist the Artist: The healthy artist displays a certain amount of grandiosity, pomposity, self-involvement, self-absorption, preoccupation with self, and an obsessive investment in perfectionism. However, this does not interfere with the artist's creative process or ability to have healthy object relations ("aesthetic survival"). The pathological artist functions at the extreme end of pathological narcissism and is dominated by such defenses as envy, control, competition, and domination, where winning becomes more pervasive than the joy of the creative process.

Narcissistic Personality: These individuals are dominated by omnipotence, grandiosity, and exhibitionist features. They become strongly invested in others and experience them as self-objects. In order to preserve this "special" relationship with their self-objects (others), they tend to withdraw or isolate themselves by concentrating on perfection and power.

Object Relations: Object relations is a powerful theory of unconscious internal object relations in a dynamic interplay with current interpersonal experience. It examines unconscious fantasies and motivations, reflecting how a person can distort reality by projecting and identifying with bad objects. This approach to understanding intrapsychic and internal conflict—including the patient's projections, introjections, fantasies, distortions, delusions, and split-off aspects of the self—is based on how one relates and interacts with others in the external world. Klein developed the idea of pathological splitting of "good" and "bad" objects through the defensive process of projection and introjection in relation to primitive anxiety and the death instinct (based on biology).

Paranoid-Schizoid Position: The paranoid-schizoid position is a fragmented position in which thoughts and feelings are split off and projected because the psyche cannot tolerate feelings of pain, emptiness, loneliness, rejection, humiliation, or ambiguity. Klein viewed this position as the earliest phase of development, part-object functioning, and the beginning of the primitive superego (undeveloped). If the child views mother as a "good breast," the child will maintain good, warm, and hopeful feelings about the environment. If, on the other hand, the infant experiences mother as a "bad breast," the child is more likely to experience the environment as bad, attacking, and persecutory. Klein, more than any of her followers, understood the primary importance of the need for mother and the breast.

Part Objects: The first relational unit is the infant's feeding experience with the mother and relation to the breast. Klein believed the breast is the child's first possession. However, because it is so desired it also becomes the source of the infant's envy, greed, and hatred and is therefore susceptible to the infant's fantasized attacks. The infant internalizes the mother as good or bad or, to be more specific, as a "part object" (a "good breast" or "bad breast"). As the breast is felt to contain a great part of the infant's death instinct (persecutory anxiety), it simultaneously establishes libidinal forces, giving way to the baby's first ambivalence. One part of the mother is loved and idealized, while the other is destroyed by the infant's oral, anal, sadistic, or aggressive impulses. In clinical terms Klein referred to this as pathological splitting. Here a parent is seen as a function of what the parent can provide, e.g., in infancy the breast, in later life money, material objects, etc. *I only love women who have big breasts!*

Persecutory Anxiety: This is the part of the psyche that threatens and terrifies the patient. It relates to what Klein has referred to as the primitive superego, an undifferentiated state that continually warns the patient of imminent danger (often unfounded). Paranoid anxiety is a feature associated with the death instinct and is more persecutory in nature. It implies the kind of anxiety from the primitive superego that is more explosive and volatile than that from the more developed superego.

Projective Identification: This is a process whereby one splits off an unwanted aspect of the self and puts it into the object, which identifies or over-identifies with that which is being projected. In other words, the self experiences the unconscious defensive mechanism and translocates itself into the other. Under the influence of projective identification, one becomes vulnerable to the coercion, manipulation, or control of the person doing the projecting.

Psychohistory: Psychohistory does for the group what psychoanalysis does for the individual. It offers a broader perspective from which to view cross-cultural differences. Using psychoanalytic tools and concepts, psychohistory allows a better understanding of individuals, nations, governments, and political events—very much as a therapist analyzes the couple as a symbolic representation of a political group or nation (DeMause 2002a, 2002b, 2006a).

Reparation: The desire for the ego to restore an injured love object by coming to terms with one's own guilt and ambivalence. The process of reparation begins in the depressive position and starts when one develops the capacity to mourn, as well as tolerate and contain the feelings of loss and guilt.

Schizoid Personality: The central features of the schizoid are the defenses of attachment, aloofness, and indifference to others. The schizoid, although difficult to treat, is usually motivated, unlike the passive-aggressive. However, because of his detachment and aloofness, the schizoid personality lacks the capacity to achieve social and sexual gratification. A close relationship invites the danger of the schizoid being overwhelmed or suffocated because intimacy may be envisioned as a relinquishing of independence. The schizoid differs from the obsessive-compulsive personality in that the obsessive-compulsive feels great discomfort with emotions, whereas the schizoid is lacking in the capacity to feel the emotion but at least recognizes the need. Schizoids differ from the narcissist in that they are self-sufficient and self-contained. They do not experience or suffer the same feelings of loss that borderlines and narcissists do. *Who, me? I don't care; I have my work, my computer, etc.*

Self Objects: This is a term devised by Heinz Kohut. A forerunner of self-psychology, the term refers to an interpersonal process whereby the analyst provides basic functions for the patient. These functions are used to make up for failures in the past by caretakers who were lacking in mirroring and empathic attunement, and had faulty responses to their children. Kohut reminds us that psychological disturbances are caused by failures from idealized objects, and that, for the rest of their lives, patients may need self objects that provide good mirroring responses.

Self-Psychology: Heinz Kohut revolutionized analytic thinking when he introduced a new psychology of the self that stresses the patient's subjective experience. Unlike with object relations, the patient's "reality" is not considered a distortion or a projection, but rather the patient's truth. It is the patient's experience that is considered of utmost importance. Self psychology, with its emphasis on the empathic mode, implies that the narcissistic personality is more susceptible to classical interpretations. Recognition of splitting and projection is virtually nonexistent among self psychologists.

Shame: Shame is a matter between the person and his group or society, while guilt is primarily a matter between a person and his conscious. Shame is the defense against the humiliation of having needs that are felt to be dangerous and persecutory. Shame is associated with anticipatory anxiety and annihilation fantasies. *If I tell my boyfriend what I really need, he will abandon me!*

Single and Dual Projective Identification: In single projective identification, one takes in the other person's projections by identifying with that which is being projected. Dual projective identification is a term I devised to describe how both partners take in the projections of the other and identify or over-identify with that which is being projected (the splitting of the ego). Thus, one may project guilt while the other projects shame. *You should be ashamed of yourself for being so needy! When you're so needy, I feel guilty!*

Splitting: Splitting occurs when a person can't keep two contradictory thoughts or feelings in mind at the same time and therefore keeps the conflicting feelings apart, focusing on just one of them.

Superego: The literature refers to different kinds of superegos. Freud's superego concerns itself with moral judgment, what people think. It depicts an introjected whole figure, a parental voice or image that operates from a point of view of morality, telling the child how to follow the rules and what happens if he or she does not. The superego deals with the "dos, don'ts, oughts, and shoulds," and represents the child's compliance and conformity with strong parental figures. Freud's superego is the internalized image that continues to live inside the child, controlling or punishing. Klein's superego centers on the shame and humiliation of having needs, thoughts, and feelings that are felt to be more persecutory and hostile in nature and invade the psyche as an unmentalized experience.

V-spot: The V-spot is a term I devised to describe the most sensitive area of emotional vulnerability that gets aroused when one partner hits an emotional raw spot in the object. It is the emotional counterpart of the physical G-spot. The V-spot is the heart of our most fragile area of emotional sensitivity, known in the literature as the archaic injury, a product of early trauma that one holds onto. With arousal of the V-spot comes the loss of sense and sensibility; everything shakes and shifts like an earthquake (memory, perception, judgment, reality).

Whole Objects: The beginning of the depressive position is marked by the infant's awareness of his mother as a "whole object." As the infant matures and as verbal expression increases, the infant achieves more cognitive ability and acquires the capacity to love the mother as a separate person with separate needs, feelings, and desires. In the depressive position, guilt and jealousy become the replacement for shame and envy. Ambivalence and guilt are experienced and tolerated in relation to whole objects. One no longer seeks to destroy the objects or the oedipal rival (father and siblings, who take mother away), but can begin to live amicably with them.

Withdrawal vs. Detachment: Detachment should not be confused with withdrawal. Withdrawal is actually a healthier state because it maintains a certain libidinal attachment to the object. When one detaches, one splits off and goes into a state of despondency. Children who are left alone, ignored, or neglected for long periods of time enter into a phase of despair (Bowlby 1969). The child's active protest for the missing or absent mother gradually diminishes and the child no longer makes demands. When this occurs, the infant goes into detachment mode or pathological mourning. Apathy, lethargy, and listlessness become the replacement for feelings of anger, rage, betrayal, and abandonment.

References

Adams, K.A. (2012). Japan: The sacrificial society. *Journal of Psychohistory*, fall.

Banner, L. (2012). Marilyn Monroe, the eternal shape shifter. *Los Angeles Times*, August 5, 2012, p. A26.

Benjamin, J. (1988). *The bonds of love: Psychoanalysis, feminism, and the problem of domination.* New York: Pantheon.

Berton, P. (1995). Understanding Japanese negotiating behavior. *ISOP Intercom* (Los Angeles: UCLA) 18(2), 1–8.

Berton, P. (2001). *Japan on the psychologist's couch.* Los Angeles: University of Southern California, Emerti Center.

Bion, W. R. (1961). *Experiences in groups and other papers.* London: Tavistock.

Bion, W. R. (1962). *Learning from experience.* London: Heinemann.

Bion, W. R. (1967). *Second thoughts: Selected papers on psycho-analysis.* New York: Jason Aronson.

Bion, W. R. (1977). *Seven servants: Four works by Wilfred R. Bion.* New York: Jason Aronson.

Bowlby, J. (1969). *Attachment and loss* (3 vols.). New York: Basic Books.

CAMFT (2002). The psychological make-up of a suicide bomber. *The California Therapist*, March/April, 14.

Carlson, J., & Sperry, L. (Eds.). (1998). *The disordered couple.* New York: Brunner/Mazel.

Carlson, J., & Sperry. L. (Eds.). (2006). *Cognitive behavior therapy of DSM-IV-TR personality disorders.* New York: Routledge.

Chambers, V. (2007). Kickboxing geishas: How modern Japenese women are changing their nation. New York: Free Press.

Coche, J. (2011). Skill loving: Couples and intimacy. Paper presented at the AGPA, January 1.

Cocks, G. (1994). *The curve of life: Correspondence of Heinz Kohut 1923–1981.* Chicago: University of Chicago Press.

Curran, D. (1996). *Tyranny of the spirits: Domination and submission in adolescent relationships.* New York: Jason Aronson.

Dallek, R. (1991). *Lone star rising: Lyndon Johnson and his times, 1908–1960.* New York: Oxford University Press.

DeMause, L. (2002a). *The emotional life of nations.* New York: Karnac Books.

DeMause, L. (2002b). The childhood origins of terrorism. *Journal of Psychohistory* 29, 340–49.

DeMause, L. (2006a). The childhood origins of the holocaust. *Journal of Psychohistory* 33, 204.

DeMause, L. (2006b). If I blow myself up and become a martyr, I'll finally be loved. *Journal of Psychohistory* 33(4), 300–307.

DeMause, L. (2007). The killer mutterland. *Journal of Psychohistory* 34, 278–300.

Dicks, H. (1967). *Marital tensions: Clinical studies toward a psychological theory of interaction*. New York: Basic Books.

Doi, T. (1973). *The anatomy of dependence*. Tokyo: Kodansha International.

Durant, W., & Durant, A. (1975) *The age of Napoleon: The story of civilization*, vol.11. New York: Simon & Schuster.

Dutton, D., & Painter, S. L. (1981). Traumatic bonding: The development of emotional attachments in battered women and other relationships of intermittent abuse. *Victimology: An International Journal* 6, 139–55.

Endleman, R. (1989). *Love and sex in twelve cultures*. New York: Psychic Press.

Evans, M. (2010). Narcissism understood: Dr Jekyll and Mr. Hyde—The personality disorder that destroys relationships, families and lives. Radio program, May 28, 2010.

Fairbairn, W. R. D. (1940). Schizoid factors in the personality. In *Psychoanalytic Studies of the Personality* (pp. 3–27). London: Routledge & Kegan Paul.

Fonagy, P., & Bateman, A. (2006). Progress in the treatment of the borderline personality disorder: Mechanisms of change in mentalization-based treatment of borderline personality disorder. *British Journal of Psychiatry* 188, 1–3.

Freud, S. (1905). *An analysis of a case of hysteria*. Standard Edition, vol. 7, pp 7–122. London: Hogarth Press.

Freud, S. (1908). Creative writers and day-dreaming. Standard Edition, vol. 9, pp. 141–53). London: Hogarth Press.

Freud, S. (1909/1955). Notes upon a case of obsessional neurosis. Standard Edition, vol. 10, pp. 153–318. London: Hogarth Press.

Freud, S. (1914/1957). On narcissism: An introduction. Standard Edition, vol. 14, pp. 69–102. London: Hogarth Press.

Freud, S.(1920/1955). *Beyond the pleasure principle*. London: Hogarth Press.

Freud, S. (1921/1979). Group psychology and the analysis of the ego. Standard Edition, vol. 18, pp. 65–143. London: Hogarth Press.

Freud, S. (1923). *The ego and id*. New York: Norton.

Frost, J. (2010). Quoted in Jonathan Burwell Frost's *The Sayings of Napoleon*. Napoleon on Woman. www.newfoundations.com/WOMAN/Napoleon.html, accessed August 19, 2011.

Fruzzetti, Alan (2006). *The high conflict couple: A dialectic behavior therapy guide to finding peace, intimacy, and validation*. Oakland, CA: New Harbinger.

Gay, P. (1988). *Freud: A life for our times*. New York: Norton.

Gilmore, D. (2001). *Misogyny: The male malady*. Philadelphia: University of Pennsylvania Press.

Giovachini, P. (1993). *Borderline patients, the psychosomatic focus and the therapeutic process*. Northvale, NJ: Jason Aronson.

Giovachini, P. (1983). *Psychoanalysis of character disorders and the study of ego adaptation*. New York: Jason Aronson.

Gray, J. (1993). *Men are from mars, women are from venus*. New York: HarperCollins.

Grotstein, J. (1981). *Splitting and projective identification*. New York: Jason Aronson.

Grotstein, J. (1987). Meaning, meaningless, and the "black hole." Self and international regulation as a new paradigm for psychoanalysis and neuroscience: An introduction. Unpublished manuscript.

Grotstein, J. (1993). Boundary difficulties in borderline patients. In L. Bryce Boyer & Peter Giovacchini (Eds.), *Master clinicians: On treating the regressed patient* (pp. 107–42). Northvale, NJ: Jason Aronson.

Grotstein, J. (2002). Personal communication.

Gunderson, J. G. (1984). *Borderline personality disorder*. Washington, DC: American Psychiatric Press.

Hall, C. S., & Nordby, V. (1999). *A primer of Jungian Psychology*. New York: Penguin.

Hayes, S. C., Strosahl, K. D., & Wilson, K. G. (2012). *Acceptance and commitment therapy*. New York: Guilford Press.

Highland, V. (2012). Personal communication.
Isay, J. (2008). *Walking on eggshells: Navigating the delicate relationship between adult children and parents.* New York: Doubleday/Flying Dolphin Press.
Johnson, F. (1994). *Dependency and Japanese socialization: Psychoanalytic and anthropological investigations into amae.* New York: New York University Press.
Kaiman, J. (2012). Lin Inspires China—to a Point. *Los Angeles Times*, February 24.
Kernberg, O. (1975). *Borderline conditions and pathological narcissism.* New York. Jason Aronson.
Kernberg, O. (1976). *Object relations theory and clinical psychoanalysis.* New York: Jason Aronson.
Kernberg O. (1985a). *Borderline conditions and pathological narcissism.* New York: Jason Aronson.
Kernberg, O. (1985b). *Internal world and external reality: Object relations theory applied.* New York: Jason Aronson.
Kernberg, O. (1991). Sadomasochism, sexual excitement, and perversion. *Journal of the American Psychoanalytic Association* 39, 333–62.
Kernberg, O. (1992). *Aggression in personality disorders and perversions.* New Haven, CT: Yale University Press.
Kernberg, O. (1995). Love relations. Normality and pathology. New Haven, CT: Yale University Press.
Kernberg, O. (1998). *Love relations: Normality and pathology.* New Haven, CT: Yale University Press.
King, L. (2012). Afghan woman slain in "latest case of domestic violence." *Los Angeles Times*, January 13.
Kivy, P. (2011). *The Possessor and the possessed: Handel, Mozart, Beethoven, and the idea of musical genius.* New Haven, CT: Yale University Press.
Klein, M. (1927). Criminal tendencies in normal children. *International Journal of Psychoanalysis* 42, 4–8
Klein, M. (1948). Mourning and its relation to manic states. In *Contributions to psychoanalysis. 1921–1945.* London: Hogarth Press. (Original work published in 1921.)
Klein, M. (1957). *Envy and gratitude.* New York: Basic Books.
Klein, M. (1975). Love, guilt, and reparation. In R. E. Money-Kyrle (Ed.), *The writings of Melanie Klein*, Vol. 1, *Love, guilt and reparation and other works, 1921–1945* (pp. 306–43). New York: Free Press. (Original work published 1937.)
Klein, M. (1984). Narrative of a child analysis. In R. E. Money-Kyrle (Ed.), *The writings of Melanie Klein*, Vol. 4. New York: Free Press. (Original work published in 1961.)
Kobrin, N. (2010a). Personal communication.
Kobrin, N. (2010b). *The banality of suicide terrorism: The naked truth about the psychology of Islamic suicide bombings.* Dulles, VA: Potomac Books.
Kobrin, N., & Lachkar, J. (2005). The she bomber symposium, September 9 http://www.frontpagemag.com.
Kobrin, N., & Simms, N. (2008). Jihadism: Parallels between autism and terrorism. *Mentalities/Mentalités* 22(2), 1–47.
Kohut, H. (1971). *The analysis of the self.* New York: International Universities Press.
Kohut, H. (1977). *The restoration of the self.* New York: International Universities Press.
Lachkar, J. (1985). Narcissistic/borderline couples: Theoretical implications for treatment. *Dynamic Psychotherapy* 3(2), 109–27.
Lachkar, J. (1986). Narcissistic/borderline couples: Implications for mediation. *Conciliation Courts Review* 24(1), 31–43.
Lachkar, J. (1991). Primitive defenses in the Persian Gulf. Unpublished paper presented at the International Psychohistorical Association, John Jay College, New York.
Lachkar, J. (1992). *The narcissistic/borderline couple: A psychoanalytic perspective on marital conflict.* New York: Brunner/Mazel.
Lachkar, J. (1993a). Paradox of peace: Folie à deux in marital and political relationships. *Journal of Psychohistory* 20(3), 275–87.
Lachkar, J. (1993b). Political and marital conflict. *Journal of Psychohistory* 22(2), 199–211.

Lachkar, J. (1997). Narcissistic/borderline couples: A psychodynamic approach to conjoint treatment. In J. Carlson & L. Sperry (Eds.), *The disordered couple* (pp. 259–82). New York: Brunner/Mazel.

Lachkar, J. (1998a). *The many faces of abuse: Treating the emotional abuse of high-functioning women.* Northvale, NJ: Jason Aronson.

Lachkar, J. (1998b). *Aggression and cruelty in cross-cultural couples*. Paper presented at the Psychohistory Congress, Paris, July.

Lachkar, J. (2000). Slobodan and Mirjana Milosevic: The dysfunctional couple that destroyed the Balkans, unpublished paper.

Lachkar, J. (2001). Narcissism in dance. *Choreography and Dance: An International Journal* 6, 23–30.

Lachkar, J. (2002c). The psychological make-up of a suicide bomber. *Journal of Psychohistory* 29(4): 349–67.

Lachkar, J. (2004a). Women who become undone: The many faces of abuse, review by Aimee Lee Ball. *Oprah Magazine*, September, pp. 300–305, 327.

Lachkar, J. (2004b). *The narcissistic/borderline couple: New approaches to marital therapy.* 2nd ed. New York: Taylor and Francis.

Lachkar, J. (2007). The psychopathology of terrorism: A cultural "V"-spot. (Forthcoming, to be published in the *Journal of Psychohistory.*) From a paper presented at the International Psychohistorical Association, June 2005, New York University.

Lachkar, J. (2008a). *The V-spot: Healing the "V"ulnerable spot from emotional abuse*. New York: Roman and Littlefield.

Lachkar, J. (2008b). *How to talk to a narcissist*. New York: Taylor and Francis.

Lachkar, J. (2008c). Psychopathology of terrorism. Paper presented at Rand Corporation, 3rd Annual Conference Terrorism and Global Security, May 9, Santa Monica, California.

Lachkar, J. (2009). How to talk to a borderline. *The therapist.* California Association for Marriage and Family Therapists (CAMFT), San Diego.

Lachkar, J. (2011). *How to talk to a borderline*. New York: Taylor and Francis.

Lawson, C. (2002). *Understanding the borderline mother: Helping her children transcend the intense, unpredictable, and volatile relationship*. Northvale, NJ: Jason Aronson.

Lewis, J. (1926). *The Bible unmasked.* New York: Forethought.

Linehan, M. M. (1993a). *Cognitive behavioral treatment of borderline personality disorder*. New York: Guilford Press.

Linehan, M. M. (1993b). *Skills training manual for treating borderline personality disorder.* New York: Guilford Press.

Los Angeles Times (2006a). Moussaoui has seldom acted in his best interests, April 17, p. A5.

Los Angeles Times (2006b). Life of a terrorist: Seeking, and finding, his jihad, April 24, p. A4.

Los Angeles Times. (2011a). North Korean leader dies: Kim enjoyed gourmet food as nation starved, December 19, A5.

Los Angeles Times (2011b). TV gets in bed with cheaters, Calendar, December 28, D1, D15.

Los Angeles Times (2012). Saying "I don't," Calendar, January 20, D1.

Lyne, A. (1987). *Fatal Attraction*, Paramount Pictures.

Mahari, A. J. (2008). Borderline personality: The quiet acting in borderline and the silent treatment. http://borderlinepersonality.typepad.com/my-weblog/2008/07/borderline-pe-2.html.

Mahari, A. J. (2009). The borderline dance and the non-borderlines' dilemma. www.aspergeradults.ca.

Mahler, M. S., Pine, F., & Bergman, A. (1975). *The psychological birth of the human infant.* New York: Basic Books.

Martin, P., & Bird, H. M. (1959). Marriage patterns: The "lovesick" wife and the "cold sick" husband. *Psychiatry*, 242–46

Masaaki, Imai. (1981). 16 ways to avoid saying no. *The Nihon Keizai Shimbun (Japan Economic Journal).*

Mason, P. (1998). Stop walking on eggshells: Taking your life back when someone you care about has a borderline personality. Oakland, CA: New Harbinger.

Masterson, J. (1981). *The narcissistic and borderline disorders: An integrated developmental approach*. New York: Brunner/Mazel.

McDougall, J. (1995). *The many faces of Eros: A psychoanalytic exploration of human sexuality*. London: Free Association Books.

Meltzer, D. (1967). *The psycho-analytic process*. London: Heinemann.

Miller, M. (2012). Serious side of making people laugh. *Los Angeles Times*, January 26, pp. D13.

Miyamoto, M. (1994). *Straitjacket society: An insider's irreverent view of bureaucratic Japan*. Tokyo: Kodansha International.

Orange County Register (2010). New charges will keep molester in prison, by Rachannee Srisavasdi and Larry Welborn, March 11.

Prager, D. (1997). *Happiness is a serious problem: A human nature repair manual*. New York: HarperCollins.

Rinaldi, R. (2012). Personal communication.

Roan, S. (2009). Trying to weather the storm: Finally, hope for those with borderline personality disorder. *Los Angeles Times*, pp. A1.

Rule, A. (2000). *The stranger beside me*. Revised ed. New York: New American Library/ Penguin Putnam.

Seinfeld, J. (1990). *The bad object: Handling the negative therapeutic reactions in psychotherapy*. Northvale, NJ: Jason Aronson.

Spencer, R. (2007). The politically incorrect guide to Islam (and the Crusades). new York: Regnery.

Sperry, L. (2006). *Cognitive behavior therapy of DSM-IV-TR personality disorders*. 2nd ed. New York: Routledge.

Stern, A. (1938). Psychoanalytic investigation and therapy in the borderline group of neurosis. *Psychoanalytic Quarterly* 7, 467–89.

Stone, M. H. (1990). *The fate of borderline patients: Successful outcome and psychiatric practice*. New York: Guilford Press.

Stoning of Soraya (2009). Directed by Nowrasteh and Stephen McEveely, Produced by John Shepherd and Todd Burns, Screenplay, Betsy Nowrasteh and Cyrus Nowrasteh, Sweden June, 2009.

Strozier, C. (2011). *Until the fires stopped burning*. New York: Columbia University Press.

Thorsen, M. (2010). The relationship between personality organization and the capacity for intimacy in adults. Dissertation, Chicago School of Professional Psychology.

Tomalin, C. (2011). *Biography of Charles Dickens*. New York: Penguin.

Tuch, R. (2000). *The single woman and the married man syndrome*. Northvale, NJ: Jason Aronson.

Turan, T. (2012). A dynamic lifting of the veil in Iran, *A Separation*, movie review.

Trowbridge, M. (2009). Powerful woman, crushed wife. www.MarthaTrowbridgeRadio.org.

Trzepacz, P. T., & Baker, R. W. (1993). *The psychiatric mental status examination*. Oxford: Oxford University Press.

Vaknin, S. (2007). *Obsessive-compulsive personality disorder (OCPD)*. Posted on the Internet, March 26.

Vaknin, S. (2011). Schizoid Personality Disorder, 216 videos uploaded by Sam Vaknin, April 26. www.youtube.com/watch?v=vu802wwef.

Vaknin, S., & Rangelovska, L. (Eds.) (2007). *Malignant self love: Narcissism revisited*. Czech Republic: Narcissus.

Vitz, P. (2010) christianpsych.org/wp_scp/category/paul-vitz/. accessed January 24, 2010.

Wallerstein, J., Lewis, J., & Blakeslee, S. (2000). *The unexpected legacy of divorce: A twenty year landmark study*. New York: Hyperion.

Winnicott, D. W. (1965). *The maturational process and the facilitating environment*. New York: International Universities Press.

Winnicott, D. W. (1971). Playing and reality. New York: Basic Books.

Index

About the Author

Joan Lachkar, PhD, is a licensed marriage and family therapist in private practice in Sherman Oaks, California. She is an affiliate member of the New Center for Psychoanalysis and the author of *The Narcissistic/Borderline Couple: Psychoanalytic Perspective on Marital Treatment*, *The Many Faces of Abuse: Treating the Emotional Abuse of High-Functioning Women*, *The V-Spot*, *How to Talk to a Narcissist*, and *How to Talk to a Borderline*. Dr. Lachkar is also a psychohistorian and has published numerous articles on marital and political conflict in the *Journal of Psychohistory*, *Frontpage*, and *Family Security Matters*. Publications include "The Psychopathology of Terrorism," a paper for the Rand Corporation.

www.ingramcontent.com/pod-product-compliance
Ingram Content Group UK Ltd.
Pitfield, Milton Keynes, MK11 3LW, UK
UKHW012039150926
475560UK00001B/89

9 780765 709097